THE
sex diaries
PROJECT

What We're Saying about
What We're Doing

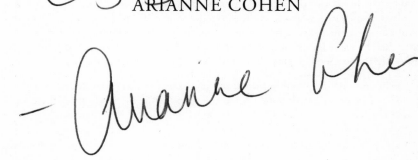

ARIANNE COHEN

WILEY

John Wiley & Sons, Inc.

A dare:
If you are in public right now, please make sure that everyone around you can see what you're reading. They're interested too. Promise.

Contents

PART THREE
poly

introduction

A FEW TANTALIZING WORDS FROM YOUR SEX DIARIES EDITOR

> We all like to know other people's secrets so we can live with our own.
>
> —Jonathan Ames

I have the best job in America. I collect sex diaries. Dozens per week, filled with love and lust and pining and people who say things like, "I'm leaving you, but when my mom calls, will you pretend that I'm still here?" It's on par with eating ice cream for a living.

You probably grabbed this book because of the word *sex*. You've chosen well: *The Sex Diaries Project* is a life-changing read, and the pages ahead will open your eyes to what is *actually* happening behind bedroom (and kitchen, bathroom, and closet) doors nationwide, in enticing bite-size portions. Yes, you will read a great amount of sex in this book in ways that will keep you riveted. But the diaries are a phenomenon because they are about all the ways that people just like you connect with—and disconnect from—others: emotionally, romantically, physically. Relationships are the centerpiece of our lives, yet rarely do we see the available options or have a context to which we can compare ourselves.

I began the project in 2007 on a personal mission: I wanted to know how to have a happy private life. At the time I was in my late 20s (single, pining), with a relationship attitude best described as stoic acceptance. But how does one learn to have a smart, fulfilling love life? Private lives, by definition, take place behind closed doors, cloaking the many clever ways that others handle their erotic lives. I thought a lot about this. My education, up to that point, had been inspired: I'd attended top schools, trained under an Olympic coach, and written for some of the country's best editors. And yet my main information on sex and relationships came from friends and . . . Vivid Videos?

This book is a tonic to that. I am thrilled to present the pages ahead, in which you can wade into the minds behind a wide array of happy bedrooms and pilfer freely. Whether you're happily married or decidedly celibate, this is your first chance to gain context for your sex and relationship urges, and grab ideas. Stealing is strongly encouraged. Much of chapters 3–6 are about this; there's a cheat sheet at the end of the book. I've structured the pages ahead so that you can spelunk through the diaries as you choose, and also pop up to read the chapter essays as they intrigue you.

I assumed that I would publish the tonic, and move on to another project. But American bedrooms are nothing if not captivating, and three years in, something miraculous happened: I was sitting on my office floor one evening, surrounded by hundreds of shreds of paper, arranging the sex diaries for this collection. I had noticed years earlier that some diarists' relationships differed vastly from others—the *way* that diarists interacted with their partners was sometimes so dissimilar that comparing two marriages was like comparing apples to donuts: both are spherical sweet foods, yes, but otherwise . . . different. And so on a whim, I grouped my shreds of paper by the *type* of relationship the diarist was in. And suddenly, patterns emerged—first in diarists' sexual escapades, and then throughout their relationships and lives. I stayed up all night rereading my database of diaries.

I realized that I was sitting on a trove: Couples I found, relate to each other in three main ways, based on their shared relationship priorities. Those priorities, in turn, forecast their whole future: their sex life, friends, family, financial status, happiness, *everything*. It's predictable, and fairly obvious in real-time relationship accounts, from the perspective *of inside* of people's minds. It was like finding a magic key.

Now, let's talk about you. Why are you holding this book? Because you're wired to. Evolutionarily speaking, your curiosity in your neighbor's bedrooms is natural. "The brain is built for love," says biological anthropologist Helen Fisher. "Those who didn't love never had children and died out, leaving people on the planet who are very interested in love." And until a few thousand years ago, humans knew a lot about their neighbors. If your fellow hunter-gatherer could only climax while donning a zebra-fur loincloth and screaming unsweet nothings, you knew about it. Now we only know what we accidentally hear through the walls, which is an odd, alienating, and misleading state of affairs. Reading *The Sex Diaries Project* is the equivalent of sitting around the campfire, learning equally about others and ourselves. It's fascinating to flip ahead and see what may be coming down the pike for you, or to read a sex diarist similar to an ex and gain new perspective.

I too began my flirtation with the sex diaries based on the word "sex," when I snagged a magazine assignment four years ago. The idea was simply to capture what people were *really* pondering and experiencing in their bedrooms and relationships. I instructed the sex diarists to include all sexual and relationship thoughts, behaviors, and arousals, and to keep it brief. The article became two cover stories and a popular weekly online column. It turns out that many people want to know how to have happy private lives. Readers eagerly awaited their weekly voyeuristic peeks in tantalizing four-minute dips. You have no idea the chaos that erupted in my inbox if I ran late.

What I found in those early sex diaries was an invisible world of profound thoughts, aspirations, and experiences. Take yourself. You have spent the past week pounding the pavement, answering the phone, and hurrying around, all while contemplating thoughts that you would never tell even your best friend: perhaps your honest concerns about your partner, your masturbation habits, or your deep-rooted worry that you're unattractive and no one will ever love you. Or perhaps you've spent all week reliving Tuesday's mind-blowing sex, breath by breath. We all think these sorts of things, all day, every day.

And, until now, this world has gone unspoken, largely lived between parentheses.

Those first few hundred sex diaries overhauled how I thought about sex and relationships. As you will quickly find, all assumptions about your neighbor's bedrooms are just that—assumptions, based on your private life, not theirs. The truth is that people run their private lives with infinite variety, much of which will be news to you. A few notions to help set the context for the book:

Private lives are just like jobs. Metaphorically speaking. While many people are 9-to-5ers, some prefer to work nights, while others juggle freelance gigs from their couch. And then there's the guy you went to high school with who seems to spend his days in Guam, eating lollipops. It's a range, and you can learn from all of them. Your experiences and fantasies are only a tiny slice of the options.

You can build whatever world you would like for yourself. Single and long-term coupledom are not the only relationship options. Relationships have infinite potential shapes, and scarcity is a myth—there are plenty of people who will love you, romantically or platonically, simultaneously or not. You can build the miniature kingdom you'd like—to meet *your* needs. Perhaps you would like one partner to stare dreamily at you for the next 50 years, with once-a-week sex. Or perhaps you're content alone, but would like periodic no-strings-attached sex. Or perhaps you want kids, and sex is secondary. They're all in the pages ahead. Some diarists prefer one-stop shopping; some don't. What's so exciting about creating your own private life is that it's up to you.

It is only by witnessing others' behavior that you gain permission to do it yourself. I should know. When I began editing the sex diaries, dating ranked in my life alongside dental appointments and taxes. Thousands of diaries later, I've shifted to a much more fulfilled existence, pretty much based only on the influence of sex diarists who exposed me to options and outlooks that I otherwise never would have considered. I was particularly mesmerized to find diarists living quite stably in relationship structures that I previously hadn't known existed, far away from the dating-commitment-marriage-children-forever escalator that many of us were raised on. You set the tone of your relationships. And you'll know what tone you like when you see it. In a sex diary.

About *The Sex Diaries Project*

I am often asked whether *The Sex Diaries Project* is a mirror of relationships and sexuality in America. Good heavens no. I have included primarily sex diarists in healthy relationships, and this is a collection, *not* a statistical survey. The sex diaries are valuable in creating a 360° view of relationships and sexuality from the inside, exploring how diarists experience their relationships, from an individual perspective. This book has more in common with the first-person narrative work of Anna Deveare Smith and Studs Terkel than, say, the sexual survey work of Alfred Kinsey. Every decade or so, a new tome of sexual behavioral statistics arrives. First from Kinsey, and later from Masters and Johnson, among many others, and most recently, the remarkable *General Social Survey* at the University of Chicago, which provides among the most varied and detailed available figures. But Kinsey himself said that you can't measure love. He knew perfectly well that sexual statistics ignore the deep (and not-so deep) urges that drive the very acts he studied. Without context—a true understanding of someone's relationship life—a sexual act has no meaning. My aim is to mine that meaning, creating a longitudinal portrait of contemporary relationship lives, which, along with sexdiariesproject.com, allows readers around the world to explore their options.

People often ask how I know that the sex diaries are real. This book joins sister *Sex Diaries Project* books the in U.K. and Italy, and continues as a journalism project, with truth as its driving mission. Though I cannot personally witness the sex diarists' experiences (and my doe eyes are quite content with this state of affairs), my frequent phone conversations with diarists confirm and elaborate details, and all diarists' circumstances are vigorously fact checked. Above all, there is no incentive to lie in an anonymous sex diarying project. The pay-off is a faithful view of one's own self. And I invite you, while you read, to go through the same process that the diarists went through, and keep your own anonymous diary at sexdiariesproject.com.

All the words you see ahead are those of the sex diarists, with the exception of minor wording adjustments for clarity. I do edit for length, because the diarists have *a lot* to say. The sex diaries are anonymous, but any fact that remains here is accurate. I have at times made details more vague, such as referring to a "bakery owner" as a "shop owner" or "small-businessman," and simply omitting the names of towns and establishments, and of course, changing all names.

The sex diaries are not all flowers and daffodils. I am always provoked by the number of men who display a level of disrespect and outright misogyny toward women that appears to be normalized in their communities and deep-rooted in their minds; I am also endlessly dazed by how often the diarists assume their partners know exactly what they want. (Let's say it all together now: Humans are not mind readers. Unless directly informed, they're rather clueless.) But overall, the sex diaries are a joyous celebration of the diversity of sexuality and relationships.

Key Observations from the 1,500 Diaries behind this Book

1. The Secret to Happiness

The happiest sex diarists share two commonalities:

- They know what their needs are (emotional, sexual, and logistical).
- They feel they are on the path to getting them met.

Whether those needs are *actually* met matters less than you may think. Perhaps a single diarist has just joined a hiking club to meet potential new partners, or agrees to six months of marriage counseling after years of fighting. What matters is that the diarist feels that she is on the right track.

Unhappy diarists know that they're unhappy—yet often have no idea what their needs are, and thus tend to be full of angst. These diarists often blame their partners, assuming they're with the wrong person, or that there's a trust issue; or they blame their relationship status, lamenting a prolonged divorce or their forever-single standing. (I assure you that your relationship status, no matter how devastating it may be, is not what ails you.) The happiest diarists approach their lives with an attitude of personal responsibility: "Okay, I have a great life or partner, but obviously some of my needs aren't getting met here."

The happiest sex diarists also share a third trait: They structure their romantic relationships in a way that best supports their needs and their connection. For some, that means marriage and cohabitation; for others, that means seeing each other twice a month for years on end. There are no rules.

2. Monogamy Is Less Common Than You Think

The goal of monogamy is common—approximately 80 percent of the sex diarists intend to enter long-term monogamous relationships. But the sex diaries capture what people are doing at any one moment. And the great irony of monogamy is that many diarists spend years of their life practicing stringent nonmonogamy while looking for "the one," overlapping casual and serious partners. Current monogamists make up just less than half of this book, with the remainder filled by diarists with zero lovers or multiple lovers.

It is not unusual for monogamous diarists to spend a third or more of their adult lives out of partnership; 43 percent of American adults are unmarried. A very large minority spends vast swaths of their life in a state that has, up to now, been defined as some amorphous form of singleness or dating.

There is an entire genre of self-help literature aimed at helping people reach and stay in two-person monogamous relationships. But many diarists are spending substantial periods of time alone by choice, or balancing multiple partners, so why not discuss that in terms that portray reality? In fact, let's do that right now.

3. Sex Diarists Come in Three States of Relationships: Solo, Partnered, and Poly

Sex diaries capture how diarists *experience* relationships, and make clear that it is pivotal to view the time period between committed relationships on its own terms. Diarists refer to these years with overtones of sex: "dating" or "playing the field" or "hooking up." Which is a mistake, because it confuses sex with relationship. The three states are distinguished by how they are meeting their needs:

Solo: A diarist meeting his or her (sexual, emotional, logistical) needs through a combination of friends and/or lover(s), and themself. A Soloist may or may not be having sex; the common denominator is not having a primary partner.

Partnered: A coupled diarist, getting his or her needs met through a relationship with a primary partner.

Poly: More than one. A subcategory, where diarists meet their needs through multiple partnerships at once. The defining factor is engaging in multiple, overlapping relationships.

Note that these are states of mind—the sex diaries take the perspective of *inside* a person's mind, and as you'll soon read, diarists' psychological transitions in and out of partnerships take place on a timeline separate from their pairings and breakups. Chapter 2 includes two diarists who are many months into a relationship, yet still meeting all of their own needs; Chapter 6 examines diarists who are still experiencing relationships that have, from the outside, ceased.

Referring to soloism on its own terms removes the nagging need to label people based on their sexual ties, while also negating much of the inherent pressure on diarists to get into a relationship. Terms like "bachelor" or "dating" all imply an assumed later partnership, which leads numerous diarists into a cycle of self-hatred and inadequacy. As you'll see in Chapter 1, some soloists have no intention of ever entering partnership.

4. Relationships Are Not Static

The diarists ahead are, at their core, a series of people moving in and out of emotional and sexual bonds over time. Partners come and go—some with half-century pit stops, some not. All partnerships end. It's a flow. Diarists constantly toss around "forever" and "one and only," but when you read the sex diaries all together, you see that they are experiencing something much more fluid. The diarists who are aware of this fare better in their breakups.

Why are relationships not static? I have, over the years, commissioned repeat diaries. Diarists rarely change, often handing in diaries that are near carbon copies. But their needs do change, sometimes quite dramatically. The same diarist who was oh-so compatible years ago with her spouse may still be compatible, but the needs of one or both have shifted radically. Even in the most stable of relationships, sex diarists' needs and wants are constantly evolving, and the happiest diarists are aware of this.

5. Age Is Just a Number

The sex diaries ahead are organized blindly to age and sexuality, for the very good reason that what body parts a diarist possesses, or how many gray hairs, has very little to do with how he or she relates to others. Age and sexuality (and, for that matter, education, race, and kids) are important in narrowing who one is attracted to. As sociologist Eva Illouz puts it, "In order to create moments of pure bonding, two people need to be in harmony together. Such harmony of the hearts is quite often a social harmony, predicated on common cultural and social references." Which is why sex diarists so often choose partners of similar race, age, class, and ethnicity. For the purposes of this book, any comments that I make apply to both heterosexual and homosexual relationships.

For me, the experience of taking up temporary residence in thousands of minds has been life altering. Whether you simply flip through the book, become an online diarist at SexDiariesProject.com, or memorize every word, you will be inspired by one of the many ways that people come together and share their souls and bodies. Or perhaps you'll transform from a foggy sense of sexuality to a more enlightened orientation. If you're not happy with where you are, a flip through *The Sex Diaries Project* may well give you a whole new game plan. Or at least a good night.

Books like this one hit nerves. You're about to read many sex diarists who made very different choices than your own. Every time you feel a wince, examine that feeling. You might find that you like the sting.

PART ONE

solo

1

dalliancing

I'M ENJOYING MYSELF

A lot of people are afraid to say what they want.
That's why they don't get what they want.

—Madonna

Some diarists are extremely good at being solo. You know these people in your own life: the friends who come out of a relationship and they seem, well, fine. And years later, after they've been playing the field for a while and nothing sticks, they're self-contained and, well, fine. That's because they are fine. The first Diarist in this chapter could be their mascot. "I must say, I have plenty of love all around me," she writes. "My family, exes, my crushes, dates. I do what I want. I am the love of my life, and it feels *really* good."

I point this out because every day, I read soloists who are fixated on the fact that they want a partner, and don't have one. Rest assured, most soloists who want a partner eventually find a great partner. But it typically takes years; longer if their personality and relationship needs are a rarer match. In the meantime, the reality is that many diarists spend their teens, twenties, and (among certain demographics) thirties primarily solo, pausing for a few years here or there in relationships; not to mention the years spent alone later in life after a divorce or the passing of a partner. Throughout their many solo years, they still need to fulfill the sexual, emotional, and financial needs that previous partners once met. Being alone truly is the default state, returned to again and again. And so this chapter looks at soloism on its own terms, not as a setback, but as a frequent and normal state of being where diarists happily meet their own needs, and engage in dalliances with others when it makes sense.

This happy solo concept tends to confuse people. While I was writing this book, I read a *New York Times* article about the CEO of Zappos, Tony Hsieh. His friend told the reporter that Hsieh "has a lot of close friends and he loves a lot of people." The reporter inquired about this and Hsieh, to his credit, replied: "I don't usually define dating or not dating. I prefer to use the term 'hang out.' And I hang out with a lot of people, guys and girls. I don't really have this one person I'm dating right now. I am hanging out with multiple people, and some people I hang out with more than others."

Let me summarize: He's a soloist. He likely had sexual ties with more than one person, but that's really not the point; he was fundamentally meeting all of his own emotional, sexual, and daily needs, in the combination of his choosing. He may be a soloist forever, or not. His relationship status was confusing to the reporter only because she was looking at it in terms of sex. And sex is just one of many needs that relationships can fulfill.

Every diarist in this chapter is sexually active and loosely seeking a relationship partner. So why are they solo in the first place? Because of their priorities. They either want to continue meeting their own needs, or their personality/sexuality/relationship priorities are more selective. In the diaries ahead, it's quite obvious which diarists will likely remain solo for the longest: The Photographer seeks a partner with a specific constellation of personality traits to fuel a relationship of intellectual and sexual exploration, which will probably take her a while to find; The Pretty Mom seems to fall in love with any man who walks slower than she does, so she'll likely transition into Partnership imminently. Whether or not diarists find partners is a fairly predictable game of numbers.

It's also a predictable game of nonmonogamy. Every diarist in this section is a monogamist, and yet their path to finding a monogamous partner is the precise opposite: rampant, nonmonogamy. Overlapping is the norm. Despite this, soloists spend most nights alone. They can easily rack up a handful of lovers in a few months and dozens of flirtations and kisses yet point to consistently empty beds. Cohabitating diarists later in the book have much more sex, because it's fairly easy to get laid when sharing a bed. Soloists have more variety. We begin in a happily empty bed in suburban Detroit

The Photographer Home for the Summer, Breaking Hearts

35, Suburban Detroit, Michigan

SATURDAY

9:00 a.m.: I've temporarily moved back home following a stint on reality TV. I am currently *very* single, though my biggest fear is that because I'm happy and not looking, someone will find me and I'll end up settling down in my hometown. Oh, no no no!

10:00 a.m.: Facebooking gorgeous guy from the TV show. I Internet-stalked him after I got the boot from the show, which required a lot of craft as I didn't know his last name. Not sure what I am expecting, as we live in different states.

3:00 p.m.: Off to a photography class I'm taking. I love being single. I have all sorts of interesting trysts that my partnered friends don't.

8:30 p.m.: Went to a party with Brian, a guy from my class, and we made out. I've also developed a crush on Jake, a coworker at my new waitressing job, and he is attractive and tall like me and much younger. Eleven years younger. His casual touches are electric.

8:32 p.m.: It should be noted that my best relationship was with a man a decade younger. It was a year of good sex, we enjoyed each other's company, and he inspired me creatively.

10:15 p.m.: Home. I love living with my mom and sister, who are rad. Though I have to be much more on the down-low about masturbating and staying over at men's houses.

SUNDAY

9:06 a.m.: Trying to figure out what I want to wear on my date tonight. Nothing too sexy, as I'm not that into Brian. Staying focused on where I see myself in six months, which is in New York City with a photography job, and lots of urban men with long-term dating potential. In the meantime I want to have as much fun as I can.

10:15 a.m.: Pass a giant store called House of Bedrooms. All sorts of interesting thoughts pass through my mind.

11:00 a.m.: Waitressing. Looking at the schedule to see when Jake and I work together next. Not at all this week.

12:30 p.m.: A creepy, bald 75-year-old man at one of my tables keeps giving me the once-over in a very voyeuristic way. Creeping me out.

3:00 p.m.: Work is over, but don't want to drive all the way home and back. Decide to nap in the employee parking lot, hoping to run into Jake who works at 5.

4:30 p.m.: No Jake. Call Brian about our date plans. He wants me to come out between 7 and 8 p.m. I am annoyed.

7:00 p.m.: Killing time in my car. I suspect Brian has hepatitis B. He's been very ambiguous. He says he has antibodies but doesn't know if he had it or just had the vaccines (he travels). Decide to steal some wifi from my car. Google says it can be transmitted from making out. I AM FREAKING OUT. I AM A HYPOCHONDRIAC.

8:00 p.m.: Arrive at Brian's apartment, and we head to a wine tasting. He looks nice but not attractive to me. He's short and pudgy and poor. I don't look for stability in men. I look for ambition and wit and the ability to be taken in by the moment. I'm thinking about right now. Isn't that what the future is based on anyway?

10:00 p.m.: Talking to another guy at the wine tasting for twenty minutes. He's kinda cute, and I can tell Brian is annoyed, but doesn't come over.

3:00 a.m.: We are out at an illegal after-hours bar with three of Brian's guy friends, talking about exploits. I've always gone with whatever turns me on. I've been with girls, and in a threesome with two men. Also went through a sex-in-public phase.

3:30 a.m.: It comes out that he used to shoot drugs when he was 20 (he's now 35). I remember from Google's note that 60–80% of IV drug users have Hepatitis B. I AM FREAKING OUT. Maintain even keel.

4:00 a.m.: Brian wants me to stay over. I say NO. Will have to bring up this Hep B thing when we are both sober.

MONDAY

11:30 a.m.: Woke up with a splitting headache, said hi to Mom, took two Advil, had a glass of water, and ate a strawberry. Immediately got back into bed and masturbated while thinking about Jake. Sleep.

3:00 p.m.: Finally up with no headache. Cranky though. Brian left a voicemail making sure I got home alright.

3:15 p.m.: Thinking about how far I have come, leaving a relation-ship that was a vexing black hole. I think it was karma, a payback for my previous dating wrongs. You get what you give.

3:17 p.m.: He was a musician, and I would be so happy to see his face after he came back from traveling, even when I was furious with him. He made me joyful in a way that wasn't logical.

4:00 p.m.: Returned Brian's call, hoping for voicemail. No dice. Said I had fun (well, I sorta did). He sent me some links on new chemicals I'm working with in printing my photography. That was nice of him. I hate nice guys.

7:00 p.m.: Called my friend Jack. He was my first boyfriend when we were 16; now we're friends. Seeing what he's up to tonight. "Noth-ing." Code for "I have no money."

7:02 p.m.: I wish I had more girlfriends. All the girls I grew up with moved away, and I don't connect with many women my age.

10:00 p.m.: Saturday night and I'm watching *The Incredibles* with my mom and sister.

SUNDAY

6:24 a.m.: In the makeup room to model in a bridal show. All the women—makeup artist, hairstylists, models—are talking about what they drank last night and who they hooked up with. I don't mention that I watched a Disney film with my family.

7:00 a.m.: One of the other girls just went into the bathroom and puked. She says she has the flu. She's like 17, and is hung over and afraid to say so.

1:00 p.m.: Bored. Sitting around waiting for the show to start. I want to leave. We all look so cheesy. Hair in big curls, lots of pastels and ribbons. Everyone else thinks this looks good. For real, they do.

1:15 p.m.: Kinda regretting saying no to Brian's brunch invitation. He lives right around the corner. I don't like seeing men more than once or twice a week in the beginning. Though I'd love to get away from the lameness I'm currently experiencing.

6:00 p.m.: At the restaurant training. Alex, the tall, attractive cook, caught me looking at him and smiled.

8:00 p.m.: Pushing my coworker for info about Jake. She says he's moody and doesn't like working here. His last girlfriend was a model.

8:15 p.m.: Alex started up a conversation. I don't want to sound mean, but he's not that smart. Bummer.

9:30 p.m.: In the manager's office making my schedule for the next week. Jake next works on Tuesday. Funny, that's when I say I can work next.

MONDAY

10:00 a.m.: Facebook message from the ex-girlfriend of my black hole ex-boyfriend. She wants to know if I'm going to see him in Brazil, where she is visiting now. Says it's beautiful and I should. Life is funny. My answer: NO WAY.

10:03 a.m.: Message from Jack, apologizing for not going to the Hamtramck music festival. He says he's stressed about money. That's cool, I get it.

10:05 a.m.: I must say, I have plenty of love all around me. My family, exes, my crushes, dates. I do what I want. I am the love of my life, and it feels really good!

11:49 a.m.: Let Brian go to voicemail. It's my day off and I want to work on my photos. Don't want to think about men.

2:12 p.m.: Break to masturbate. Jake is in my head.

3:00 p.m.: More self-loving. Jake comes to mind. I've been anxious lately and this is my release. I'm afraid that I'm going to get to know him and the crush will implode. But right now the fantasy person I have created is nice.

6:15 p.m.: Finally listened to Brian's voicemail. He tried a photo technique I told him about and was happy with the results.

9:30 p.m.: Just sat and talked with Brian outside the darkroom for two hours about art, literature, screwed-up people, and strippers. Then we spent another hour in the darkroom. He helped me figure out the enlarger. I helped him choose prints. I like how his mellow vibe makes me feel.

TUESDAY

8:00 a.m.: Awake. It's those lazy moments in the morning that I miss most and long for.

8:30 a.m.: Brian emailed about hanging out with him on his birthday. I hate spending occasions with boyfriends until we are serious.

3:30 p.m.: Working a double shift. Went to a temple on my break to meditate. I'm not very thrilled with my job and everything doesn't seem so great today. It's just a bad day. Need some perspective.

5:00 p.m.: Back at work. Jake is working. Sweet. He looks cute.

7:00 p.m.: The hostess mentions that Jake and I would make super tall babies. Inappropriate, but I secretly love it. He said, "Hmmmmmm. Maybe we should try it." I laughed.

7:15 p.m.: Another server walks up and totally out of the blue says that he didn't know that Jake was dating Chrissy, a fellow server who I really like. I am bummed. And confused. Jake has been rather boldly flirting and never mentioned it.

8:03 p.m.: Still bummed by this news.

8:30 p.m.: Jake totally just gave me that sparkly eye when we passed in the hall. He and Chrissy must not be serious.

9:15 p.m.: Jake and I are in the manager's office, and without my asking, he volunteers to contact an ex of his who might be able to help get me shooting work. I like this guy.

10:02 p.m.: Standing out back, when the busboy asks when we are going out on a date. Is he serious?! He offers to walk me to my car. He's a nice *kid*.

WEDNESDAY

12:00 p.m.: Catch myself thinking about Jake. When he trained me last week, it seriously felt like we were on a date. A good one, too.

2:22 p.m.: Okay. I feel foolish that I've been thinking about my coworker and masturbating, especially now that he's dating a coworker. I feel tricked.

3:30 p.m.: This doesn't keep me from continuing to do it. Three times in one hour.

10:00 p.m.: Long talk with my mom about relationships. She thinks it's natural for older woman to date younger men, and brings up director Katherine Bigelow, and her 21-year-younger boyfriend. She also says I don't have my standards too high, and when I find the right one, I won't have to think about it. I'll just know. I love my mom.

10:13 p.m.: She also advises me to stay away from Jake, unless he has another job on the side. She's so funny. And right. ✳✳✳

How to Be a Happy Soloist

The previous and next diarists, along with the hundreds of happy soloists I've read, share a few common features:

They know what their current needs are, and they meet them. Both women have looked at their next 6–24 months, and determined which relationships would make them happy on a week-to-week basis *until* they meet their next partner: lots of friends, and when it makes sense, a casual lover. The Pretty Mom takes great glee in her online lover who obviously fills a need while she's single. The Photographer is in close contact with her vibrator. They see their solo time not as a means to an end, but a chapter in itself.

They're flexible in the many roles lovers can play in their lives. Both women build casual relationships with men they know will never be life partners. Diarists more experienced at dating are often much more open-ended in the many happy roles potential lovers and friends can play in their lives. It's the younger diarists, like The Single Virgin in the next chapter, who tend to be much more conservative in their relationship structures, prone to toeing the line of heterosexual monogamy with every potential partner, simply because it's the only path in their minds.

They fill their lives with "friend families" of interconnected friends and relatives who fulfill many of their needs. You'll see it throughout this book. The Photographer spends Saturday night watching Disney with her family; The Pretty Mom—who is still recovering from a years-old heartbreak—spends the same Saturday dancing with loose friends. There is a Buddhist concept that there is only one "right now," so it's best to enjoy it. And the diarists who enjoy their "right now," no matter how sexless or Disney-involved it may be, are contented people. It's the diarists who pine to be in someone else's arms "right now" who are miserable. "Having wonderful friends is in many ways similar to being in a relationship," writes The Pretty Mom. She is right.

The Pretty Mom with Many Suitors and a Meticulous Sexual Memory

37, Ventura County, California

SATURDAY

7:40 a.m.: Fell asleep last night thinking about Nathan, a single dad who's had a crush on me for about a year. Again. He likes me, but he's too entangled with his new divorce. Come on Nathan! I want you to be my bunny slope back into love.

7:50 a.m.: A "bunny slope" is exactly what I'm looking for. I want a practice run before getting too involved with a man again; a long-term lover who can rebuild my sexual confidence. Nathan is my first choice, although my kaleidoscope of possibilities is vast these days.

7:54 a.m.: Voicemail from Philippe. He sang me a message. Philippe was my first foray back into dating, a year ago. He smells better than any man I've ever met. He plays guitar better than anyone. Too bad he knocked up that other girl, or else we'd still be lovers. We are still dear friends. Maybe we'll be together again in 10 years or something.

9:51 a.m.: Making plans for a big dance party this evening with my friends, my weekly evening out. Being a single mom is limiting, but my mom helps me a lot since my five-year-old son's father, Carlos, is a jackass and has totally disappeared. I'm almost over that disaster, though it's hard to look into my son's eyes every day and see Carlos.

10:10 a.m.: Off to work—I'm a language teacher. I have a big crush on one of my students. He is 22 and from Switzerland. Young. Flirtatious. Hot. He looks deep into my eyes and smiles and makes me blush. I wonder if my other students notice. I have never had an affair with a student, although I have come close.

1:10 p.m.: Just finished class, and Swiss Guy tells me to give his regards to my husband. I tell him I don't have a husband, and he smiles at me slyly.

8:57 p.m.: Just dropped off my son and am getting ready. There are a few men I'd like to run into, and only one I'd like to be with: Nathan. The rest are simply too young or far from my reality. I plan to just do as I always do and have fun with whomever I connect with and dance.

2:10 a.m.: At the party. I am asked, as I always am, why I don't have a boyfriend. I look 28. I have amazing legs, great hair, nice skin, a beautiful face. The only reason I can think of is that I'm not ready. Carlos hurt me really badly. I am still recovering.

4:00 a.m.: Just home. Most definitely danced my little heart out. A Scorpio ogled me and asked me out, but he was drunk. His wife showed up after he passed out and my feelings passed quickly. Met a French boy whom my friend invited, apparently for me. He was sweet, and all over me. I had to walk away from him to leave, exhausted. I can't stop thinking about Nathan, and how I wished he was there.

SUNDAY

10:40 a.m.: I never feel better than after a night of dancing. I love the person I am when I dance: bold, flirtatious, spiritual, and sparkling.

10:46 a.m.: I check my email every morning for news of my son's father. I wish I could forget. We met as housemates while living a bacchanalian life in Europe. We were together nearly three years—it was passionate and tumultuous, with a dynamic sexual attraction like no other I've had. We lived to make love to one another. But when I got pregnant, we were breaking up. He was so angry at me for keeping the baby. I may still be in love with him. I know for sure that I think of him every day. It's too bad that I haven't heard from him in five months.

11:27 a.m.: I remember the first time we made love, after we had confessed our love for one another. We started kissing in the hallway outside of my bedroom, and he tore off my skirt and pushed me against the wall and we had sex right there in the hallway, while our other housemates slept. Then we moved into his bedroom and made love as if we'd known each other all of our lives. We kissed and touched and licked and sucked and felt and grinded every part of our body, until the next day when I had to pack my things to go back to the States. No wonder he followed me to the U.S.

3:18 p.m.: I didn't date at all for four years, save one or two one-night stands, and many close male friends. I am still recovering. The anger, at least, is gone. It wasn't until I moved here last year that I began to blossom.

7:00 p.m.: At dance party number two this weekend, with my son. It's a celebration of music and dancing, a bit of a hippie love fest. Great music. Lots of eye candy. Groovy.

10:40 p.m.: Home. A single dad named Martin was there tonight, who I had a little thing with a while back. I also met a single dad who I've seen at the park who seems nice. And the Scorpio was there. I've been having so much fun lately, giving off and getting so much sexual energy.

11:29 p.m.: Looking for El Greco online. He is my cyber lover. I'm in the mood for some cybersex with him. My friend introduced us, and he moved away before we could get to know one another. We broke each other's Internet cherries a few months back. Now it's kind of a tradition. He is so hot. Cybersex is the best masturbation ever, because you are truly not alone—you know that someone is thinking about you, you read their words, and they are doing the same thing.

MONDAY

8:24 a.m.: Son woke me up, of course. Today Philippe and his pregnant girlfriend are getting kicked out of their house around the corner. I was quite jealous at first—she got pregnant to trap him—but now it's normal to stop by their place, and I've come to enjoy them as a couple. Out of it came a very solid and beautiful friendship that has helped me grow more than most others I've had.

9:30 a.m.: Ostensibly helping Phillipe move, but really remembering my first night in bed with him. He said he wanted to know who I was before we had sex. It was so enlightening and sweet. We couldn't stop kissing.

6:07 p.m.: Sometimes I surprise myself with how brazen I can be. Two of my men are coming over right now. Single dads with daughters. Both at the same time. Lovely.

9:22 p.m.: So, that was interesting. Martin came over with his daughter, per my son's request. I'm not sure how I feel about Martin these days. Our kids get along really well. Nathan came too. We hang out pretty much every Sunday, but he is in the beginning stages of divorce.

10:38 p.m.: Bed. I'm having crazy fantasies about my Swiss student this evening. After all of the men, I'm thinking about him! He is so sexy to me. . . mmmm. I think it may be time to finally quench some of my sexual hunger that has built up from this weekend.

10:48 p.m.: I am lucky to have had some wonderful sex. I like it kind of rough. I like to be dominated. I like a man to push me against a wall and tear my clothes off. I like to be grabbed and fucked wherever we are—an elevator, on a trail, in the car. You get the picture.

TUESDAY

6:01 a.m.: Getting up this early is so difficult. Damn. With a schedule like mine, who has time for a sex life?

6:22 a.m.: Showering, thinking about when I fell in love for a few hours last month. I was visiting friends in the Bay Area, and met a guy who looked like Jakob Dylan. It was as if we were very old friends or soul mates. The energy and connection was ridiculous. We hung out for a few hours, then he walked me to my car, arm in arm, like a gentleman. He grabbed me and held me as we giggled. I was anticipating the kiss. But the kiss never came. He had been seeing someone for a month. I was stricken. I had truly thought that I had finally met someone who met all of my criteria. He kissed me slowly and sweetly on the neck as I got in my car. And that was all.

10:48 a.m.: Working. Boring so far. Feel like I'm still waking up. Not even any fantasies.

11:46 a.m.: I think that being Catholic has greatly contributed to my insatiable attraction to Jewish men. Jewish men are my fetish. Sometimes I have no idea that someone is Jewish, and find out later. That happened with Philippe.

3:42 p.m.: Oh boy. That Swiss student is undressing me with his eyes. It's clear that I'm giving back his energy, and I don't want the class to notice. But I can't help it. He has such beautiful lips. I want to be completely alone with him in the dark, to push those amazing lips into mine, tangle my fingers in his hair, and wrap my body around his. Oh, boy. This is a student I'm talking about.

5:39 p.m.: Texting Nathan. Texting makes flirting easier, much less intimidating.

8:56 p.m.: Home from a friend's birthday dinner. I love my community here. I have such a great circle of friends who really nourish me and make me happy. Having wonderful friends is in many ways similar to being in a relationship.

9:57 p.m.: I'd like to meet a certain Swiss man in the park, late at night, under a full moon. I want his hands to creep under my shirt as we kiss, perhaps pushed up against a tree in the darkness, and find my nipples. I want to feel his breath in my ear, on my cheek, on my chest. I want to run my tongue all over his body, taste his skin, smell his hair, feel his skin on my skin, longing and pressing. I want it to feel forbidden and wrong, and very exciting. I want to not be able to stop, to be swept away by uncontrolled lust. I want him to fuck me standing up, holding me up by my open legs, as he kisses me until we both orgasm.

10:13 p.m.: Actually, something very similar happened to me not long ago. I ran into a guy I'd met a couple of weeks earlier. We started talking and hung out the rest of the night and, carried away by our sexual urges, had sex in the bushes, standing up, he holding me up by my open legs. It was one of my hottest sexual experiences in years. We remained lovers for a couple of months, and then it faded.

WEDNESDAY

6:13 a.m.: Woke up thinking about Carlos. It's shocking to me that he would not want to know about his son.

9:56 a.m.: I feel blue today. I'm wondering if I will ever find love. I'm tired of meaningless sex, which is why I stopped it after my last little evening a few weeks ago. I am quite happy with all of the friendships I have with men, and the love I feel for them, but none seem to be able to commit to me. It's frustrating.

10:00 a.m.: I am only thinking of the most important man in my life today: my son. Just toured the local public kindergarten.

11:35 a.m.: Swiss student wearing glasses today. Lord help me.

2:46 p.m.: Fantasizing about another instance of brief love. Ten years ago I met a Peruvian guy in Spain. I ended up in his bed at around 2:00 a.m., and stayed until 8:00 p.m. the next day, sleeping, drinking beer, eating very little, kissing, playing guitar, talking, licking, sucking. He had these orange drapes which danced in the breeze. Honestly, I cannot remember how many times we had sex. We couldn't stop. I went home and we drifted apart. But I'll never forget those hours.

10:33 p.m.: Jeez. You'd think by all of my entries that I never sleep with Americans.

10:39 p.m.: Going to bed with memories of the Swiss smile. Tomorrow is a new day. And I have no doubt that I will find him, one day. He is out there waiting, just as I am waiting for him. . . my next fabulous, fantastic love.

· · · · · · · · · · · · · · · · · · **Diary Insight** · · · · · · · · · · · · · · · · · ·

A sex trick for you: Why does The Pretty Mom enjoy chronically good sex? Because good sex is a mind-set. Psychologist Leonore Tiefer posits that great sex requires a "symbolic investment" to provide the necessary mental spark. The Pretty Mom invests meaning into all her sexual activities, such as the one-night stand in Spain that she recasts as *Eighteen Hours with a Stranger in a Strange Land with Orange Curtains Blowing in the*

Sun. Without that infusion of meaning, the exact same sex would be ho-hum. And then there's our next diarist who does the opposite: he doesn't invest, and thus, is not particularly wowed by his encounters. . . .

. . . .

Diarists Considering Not Being Solo

The Eligible Guy and The Outdoorsy Guy answer a key question you might have: *What the heck is he thinking?* The Eligible Guy is *that* guy you know who inexplicably has a small harem. The Outdoorsy Guy is the smart, early-30s male with many admirers and commitment phobia.

First, the harem. The book's resident lothario, The Eligible Guy, is searching for a wife, a task he accomplishes through volume. He uses text messages to interact aloofly with a large number of women, and is rather extreme in his soloist refusal to allow the women in his life to meet any of his emotional needs. He is emotionally detached because he hasn't vested enough needs to a partner to warrant attachment. It's cyclic—by continually meeting his own needs, he doesn't provide his partners any way to meaningfully enter his life, so he has all the problems of partnership and few of the benefits beyond sex. He wakes up to an empty bed and writes, "I am completely dissatisfied with my personal life."

Not surprisingly, he hurts many women. His blunder is common in the diaries—he confuses honesty with responsibility. He is truthful with partners about his sexual activities, but he is not remotely honest with himself about the priorities of his partners, nor how he is emotionally affecting them. The result is crying partners. He's wielding a negative power dynamic over them.

Why are these diarists, both many months into serious relationships, in the solo chapter? Because relationships are a state of mind, and the diaries reveal that the first year of a relationship is, quite typically, not really a relationship at all in the sense of people meeting each other's needs. It's two soloists spending time together and having sex, continuing to meet their own needs. Most diarists continue ceaselessly functioning as individuals 6–12 months into serious relationships, meeting their own financial, emotional, and sexual needs. The same handholding and lovey-dovey nuzzling that, from the outside, looks like a definite partnership, is experienced on the inside as an almost staunch phase of soloism. In fact, some relationships stay in this stage forever. It's not unusual to see diarists, particularly men in their twenties and thirties, who have *never* left solo. They tend not to realize this detail.

Why is the transition from solo into Partnership so fraught? It's risky. Entrusting a partner with one's needs equates to emotional vulnerability. Translation: the breakup will be painful. Which is why solo is a state of mind that lags far, far beyond the visual signs of coupledom. It's a shift that's largely invisible from the outside, yet a universal shift in the diaries. You'll see the diarists ahead navigating three major psychological shifts, each of which have caused lesser ships to wreck:

1. Identity. The diarists are shifting from seeing themselves as individuals to one-half of a partnership.
2. Needs. Whether cooking dinner or resolving arousal, the diarists are no longer handling every need alone. Some needs fall through the cracks.
3. Priorities. The diarists are choosing their relationship priorities— and seeing whether their needs will align.

Both diarists ahead express frustration at their girlfriends, not realizing that the transition they are experiencing is largely within themselves. The Outdoorsy Guy complains repeatedly, saying he wishes he "felt more free and open" in the relationship. Whenever diarists blame their partners anywhere in this book, it's a red flag that their own needs are not getting met.

As with most diarists, sex distorts the picture. The Outdoorsy Guy is amusingly upbeat about his girlfriend in the 12 hours of each postcoital glow, writing, "This relationship is so unique! I forget how special our bond is." This is a third of the time. And yet his brain just can't quite buy that he has a girlfriend named Alyssa.

The Outdoorsy Guy Feeling the 7-Month Itch

31, Portland, Oregon

FRIDAY

11:38 a.m.: I am at work and haven't been thinking about relationships or sex today. Only about data.

11:41 a.m.: Yikes. Thinking about the fantastic little clip of lesbian porn I watched on the Internet last night. It reminded me how much I like to give cunnilingus, and at the same time, I'm reminded of how I don't really like to do that with Alyssa.

12:12 p.m.: Just got a random Gchat from Lauren, an older coworker I dated briefly. She is crazy, but I loved going down on her.

3:46 p.m.: Just got back from a walk with Lauren. Our dating ended because she just wasn't that into it. I can't say exactly why, but it had to do with her having different priorities.

4:00 p.m.: Not excited about hanging out with Alyssa tonight. This feeling is furthered when she says that all she wants to do tonight is hang out with me. We have been dating for seven months, and she moved from another state to be with me.

6:11 p.m.: Still at work, an hour later than I need to be, working and listening to music. Friday night. Lamesville.

11:00 p.m.: Had a frustrating evening with Alyssa and her roommates, hanging out and eating dinner. Alyssa and I watched a silly movie and are now going to bed. Friendly, not intimate.

SATURDAY

12:18 p.m.: Just got home from Alyssa's house. Talked a little about how I wish I felt more free and open in our relationship. She didn't say much. Most mornings she has sex on her mind, and doesn't really listen to me. (Ha.) I was sort of in the mood, so we had sex and it was fun. Mellow breakfast. Alyssa is great most of the time.

4:22 p.m.: I think of myself as being bad at relationships, like there is something I don't get. My primary issue now is my desire to have multiple casual partners, as opposed to one committed, closed relationship. Why? Because I am not fulfilled sexually in the relationship I'm in.

6:13 p.m.: Alyssa is very patient and forgiving, and has never broken up with a boy. She is a peacekeeper. Were it not for me, I imagine this relationship could last forever. It seems like I need to get over some hurdle if I am to avoid tearing this relationship down.

9:42 p.m.: On the topic of sex and other women, tonight I am pleasantly annoyed by all the uninteresting girls out with us, and content and glad to have Alyssa.

9:45 p.m.: I have an inability to date or stay in a relationship with women who are not smart, or those who cannot at least act intelligent and articulate most of the time. This is a fantastic juxtaposition to my vanity and desire for attractive women. These two things make me very picky. And an asshole.

12:30 a.m.: Fun night. Got a little drunk with friends, including Alyssa, and went to a reggae show. Broke into new territory with her. We smoked pot together. She *never* smokes and doesn't like it when I do. But we talked about it and she demonstrated an amazing ability to push her boundaries. We had some good talks, were silly.

1:00 a.m.: Fun late-night bike ride home and some pretty great sex before bed.

SUNDAY

9:15 a.m.: Woke up enjoying Alyssa's warm body and snuggles.

12:21 p.m.: She just went home. This relationship is so unique. Alyssa is so unique. It's certainly new territory, and I forget how special our bond is. Sometimes I feel like our relationship right now is not necessarily what I want, but it might be exactly what I need. I'm never quite sure what I need.

12:30 p.m.: I should say that I am happy that I am "in a relationship," as opposed to being "not in a relationship," and that my relationship is very free and open and fun and loose. However, I would prefer my status to be: "in a relationship." It seems like there's no asterisk option. If after the next several years I still haven't learned how to relax and accept an intimate relationship for what it is, I imagine I will be a curmudgeonly old bastard, all alone.

1:02 p.m.: Brief thoughts pertaining to sex with strangers: Never tried because it has always seemed wrong. Immoral. But I am growing more and more keen on the idea of going to Craigslist's Casual Encounters and meeting up with a complete stranger and acting out some sexual fantasy. I still feel like that kind of thing is not within the realm of healthy, normal people. And then there is the issue of going behind my girlfriend's back.

10:44 p.m.: Spent the evening with roommates. Two short conversations with Alyssa on the phone, of no significance. Just checking in, talking about plans. No pressure to sleep together tonight. Feels nice.

10:47 p.m.: I'm on the Internet and I will probably look at a little bit of porn. Or maybe I'll be good and just pick up a book and read till I fall asleep.

MONDAY

9:51 a.m.: Reflecting on my relationship with Lauren, then recalling several years back with Gillian. I have a fondness for these relationships that is odd, and I think what they have in common is that: 1) I liked who I was in the relationship, and 2) I didn't see the relationship really going anywhere, and neither did they necessarily. When there is pressure to "make this work," I seem to fall apart, I get grumpy, I don't really like myself as much.

11:06 a.m.: Work. I feel like I have been wandering aimlessly, doing very little in my life, not going anywhere. I realize that most people probably feel this way, like they should be doing something differently.

12:00 a.m.: Alyssa is sleeping over, and there is zero intimacy. She got a little upset and almost left because she wanted to have sex, and I was tired and not in the mood. I don't know what it is, but I am an incredibly sensual person who thinks about sex all the time, yet when it comes to having sex with my partner, I'm just not that excited.

TUESDAY

10:26 a.m.: I really like a skinny waist, with round breasts in my face. Alyssa is boxy, narrow hips, thick torso, broad shoulders.

11:17 a.m.: It's gotta be fairly common for people to just want to bone down, right? Maybe that new girl with that big ol' booty in my office is one of those.

11:19 a.m.: I hold honesty as the highest virtue. And yet today I am considering going behind Alyssa's back. Why can't I be honest with her? This is the very first relationship where an affair is even remotely possible. In all previous relationships, my faithfulness was never even close to being an issue.

4:58 p.m.: Just got back from lunch with older ex-girlfriend, Gillian. We often meet up for coffee and chat. We have become pretty good friends since our breakup two years ago. Alyssa does *not* like that we are still friends.

5:22 p.m.: I will always love Gillian. That relationship was a landmark. It was the only time I've really had my heart broken, like crushed. It's the only relationship where I was all-in, from the beginning. It was what I thought I always wanted, dream girl stuff. I value growth, and there was tons in that relationship.

6:58 p.m.: Alyssa wants me to come over to her house and give her a kiss. That doesn't really float my boat. I wish it could be a quick passionate fuck.

9:00 p.m.: Lied to Alyssa when she asked, "Oh, did you go out with your coworkers?" Even though we just got a bite to eat, and it was purely catching up, I know that she wouldn't approve. I never outright lie like that, but this is the second time now, both having to do with an ex. I hate this.

The Eligible Guy with the Pick of the Litter

29, Camden, New Jersey

THURSDAY

7:40 a.m.: Up earlier than usual, thinking about a conversation last night about how I always end up sleeping with my female friends. Girls talk to me, sleep with me, then fall for me. While these girls all tell me that they are all right with our casual relationship, they talk about me behind my back to my roommate and our mutual friends. It gets a little out of hand.

7:50 p.m.: I am in love with two women, and at least three others love me. Just so you understand: I am a handsome African-American with a master's degree. So basically, I have part of the market cornered. I get pressure from everyone to make a decision. And I just feel like I need to because I'm getting old. I'm gonna be 30. But I'll be in my next relationship for a while, and I don't wanna make a wrong decision.

7:00 p.m.: Long day at work. I work in the inner-city, usually 9–7.

8:00 p.m.: At a bar with my roommate. He has a way with relationships. It's "we're together when you're around." And his current girl lives in Maryland.

9:45 p.m.: Drinking. I think I may give in and sleep with someone tonight that I have no business sleeping with. It's Tonesha, who's still an undergrad. She's always hitting me up—"What are you doing?" "Wanna hang out?" She lives nearby. No chance I'll ever be in a relationship with her.

11:21 p.m.: Well, I am proud of myself. I could send a text and be in the midst of some passionate fulfilling sex. I'll just rub one out.

11:22 p.m.: I exist only in the gray area, in every aspect of my life, but especially in my personal life, which is utter chaos.

FRIDAY

8:39 a.m.: I am completely dissatisfied with my personal life. That is the thought I woke up to in my empty bed.

9:00 a.m.: Off to work. Thinking about how I am going to get myself into a deeper hole this weekend. My situation is weird because a lot of the girls I deal with don't live within 45 minutes of me. Monique lives in New Brunswick. And Jennifer lives in New York.

2:00 p.m.: I think I finally figured out why I can't settle down. When I see a female, the first thing that crosses my mind is, "What are my chances?"

7:22 p.m.: Just finished BBQ'ing for two hundred people at a community event. Sometimes I think I'm too busy at work to settle down—that, and helping out my family financially.

8:00 p.m.: Amanda just came over. I've been trying to withdraw from her, but she lives a couple blocks away. She asks what I'm doing, and I say nothing, so we watch a little TV. That's usually how it happens with her. It's not like we go to a romantic dinner and then make love.

10:00 p.m.: After going for pizza, I walk into an afterparty that's apparently at my house. Tonesha's here. My roommate is mutual friends with all my girlfriends, so they get invited to stuff even if I don't want them there.

10:15 p.m.: It's me and these five other dudes, and Amanda and Tonesha. And basically all the guys are playing video games, and all the girls will stay late to see who's going to leave first.

1:00 a.m.: Amanda isn't leaving. She says, "I'm drunk and I don't wanna go home." Which I probably shouldn't allow. But I have this thing where I can't say no if I'm not in a relationship. If a chance presents itself, I'll sleep with a girl. I rationalize it.

2:15 a.m.: Amanda's asleep. The sex is always pretty passionate. It's never no kissing or something. And she usually sleeps over. Their leaving isn't an option for me. And generally, the girls I sleep with, for the most part, I like in a very endearing way. Except Tonesha. She has extra-annoying friends, and doesn't think clearly about stuff, and we always get into these crazy arguments.

SATURDAY

10:14 a.m.: My married brother calls to tell me that I'm "living the life." He doesn't understand that I feel like I have four wives. I tell him to watch *Big Love*.

11:45 a.m.: Uh-oh. Voicemail from Jennifer. She called at 11:00 p.m. We first hooked up three years ago, but I was seeing my high school sweetheart, who I dated for nine years on-and-off. We reconnected six months later. She's white. Race always plays a more important role in my decisions than it should.

12:00 p.m.: State of the Relationship talk with Jennifer, which we have every two weeks. Basically, she doesn't think I give her enough detail of where we're at. I say, "I'm close to making a decision." She says, "I've been patiently waiting, and I'm sick of this," and I'm like, "You gotta do your thing," and she says, "Why don't you just break up with me?" I tell her about all of them—she knows more than any of them. She says, "At least you're honest." By the end of the conversation, she's somewhat reassured, and she loves me again.

12:02 p.m.: I'm sure everything will be fine for a few days, then something will happen again, like I won't call her, and she'll get upset. It's not like I'm ignoring her—she didn't call me! And then we'll do a State of the Relationship again.

2:00 p.m.: Train to New Brunswick to see Monique. I met Monique my senior year in class, and thought she was fascinating because she was a Latino female. Fast forward to three months ago: I'm back for grad school and we became intimate.

4:00 p.m.: Picnic in the park. Just she and I, and a long make-out session.

7:30 p.m.: We're getting a hotel room. She knows that I've slept with most of my female friends, but whether she knows I still do? Who knows? We're in the gray area, and there haven't been any parameters set.

9:00 p.m.: We just had hot sex, and I'm taking a moment to check my messages. I generally have sex as if I am making love, if that makes any sense. I rarely have bad sex.

9:10 p.m.: Really torn between Jennifer and Monique. Both are smart, attractive, and sweet. Monique's got some sass to her, and I don't get none of that from Jennifer—she's more laid back. I haven't really had the full range of sexual experiences with Monique yet, and that worries me; sex with Jennifer is satisfying, if not spontaneous. She gives very good oral—some of the best I've ever had. She could lose a pound or two here or there, but she is beautiful.

9:36 p.m.: I am what one would call a sexual thinker. I think often about sex and my sexual experience and my recent relations.

11:00 p.m.: Good night.

SUNDAY

10:22 a.m.: Train home. Other girls who are in love with me right now include: B, a law student I met through her roommate. She is definitely in love with me, and she is white. And L, who I met at school. She is African-American. She has liked me for five years. She is kinda annoying and definitely in love with me since we hooked up two years ago. And D. I met her in grad school and she is also African-American. She acts like she is not in love with me and maybe she is not, but she likes me a lot and I can have her whenever I want. Then there's my high school sweetheart. I still have some feelings for her and could have her back. We haven't hooked up in a while.

10:26 a.m.: If I don't have sex tonight, I'll rub one off to one of them.

11:34 a.m.: Heading to my cousin's birthday party. I often find myself fantasizing about older women, mid-40s.

6:00 p.m.: All day at the party. I did get this girl's number—31, African-American, lives in Philly. My cousin was trying to hook me up. If a girl gives me her number, I take it. I probably won't call her—I do that often.

11:35 p.m.: D, L, and B are all very good in bed. D and L give phenomenal oral. D is great all around. But with Jennifer there's that emotional connection. Maybe the difference is how I feel when it's over and I am looking in their eyes. It's either, "Damn, she is great in bed," or, "Damn, that was good, I love her."

MONDAY

1:07 p.m.: Work is killing me. It would be kinda cool to have sex in my office with a coworker, but my coworkers are generally unattractive.

4:00 p.m.: Graduation ceremony for my master's degree. Thinking about one of my professors. She is not attractive but she is so nice and is such a great professor. If she came to me I would probably sleep with her. Don't ask me what that means.

6:00 p.m.: Post-graduation drinks. I'm not really celebrating, but Amanda's over.

11:00 p.m.: Amanda just left. She was sitting around, waiting for me to make a move and I just didn't make one.

11:49 p.m.: Mostly I am scared that I will lose my friendships with the females I have been intimate with. Outside of the sex they provide unbelievable support. That's a big issue. An outsider could call them "ego feeders," but if you knew them, you would know they are just sweet girls. Monique, B, my high school sweetheart, and Jennifer are all awesome girls. L and D, a little less, but they have their moments.

TUESDAY

3:33 p.m.: No sex + long work hours = suicidal thoughts.

4:19 p.m.: I am an African-American and this plays a huge role in my decision-making and I hate that it does. If I decided to be with a white girl long-term, I worry about how I would be perceived in the African-American community.

6:00 p.m.: Sexting back and forth with Monique.

7:35 p.m.: Monique told me that one of her fantasies is to have sex in a store dressing room. Ever since then, I have been daydreaming about it. I imagine I am in the dressing room and I text her to pick out something sexy. She chooses a backless dress (her back is unbelievably sexy), and I grab her wrist firmly, turn her around, press her against the wall, and kiss her neck. One hand would make its way up her thigh and the other massage her breast. With the one hand I rip her pantyhose off and rub her clitoris as she rubs my penis through my pants. I would take my penis and stick it in her vagina from behind, stroking her until we both climax.

10:00 p.m.: Worked until late, then board meeting. When I'm around educated young people, there are a whole lot of opportunities for me in terms of young females. I definitely could have a lot more sex.

11:00 p.m.: Jennifer on the phone. She's upset because we didn't talk very long. But sometimes I'm really tired, and I don't feel like calling, and I don't feel like texting.

WEDNESDAY

8:00 a.m.: Decided that I'm probably not going to sleep with Tonesha and Amanda ever again. Amanda is so nice and sweet. I've gone long periods without sleeping with her. Like a month. I know she's gonna end up getting hurt, so I'm trying to withdraw.

10:15 a.m.: Text from D: "What you up to? You haven't called. I'm worried." She's upset because I don't keep in touch. I had sex with her three weeks ago, and she's told my roommate all this stuff she knew he would tell me.

1:47 p.m.: Trying to work and just got into a disagreement with Jennifer on instant messenger. She has given me plenty of opportunities to walk away. More than anything I worry about regrets. I hate regrets.

1:50 p.m.: Jennifer asks what is holding up my decisions. Is it that she's white? Is it the other girl? Or is it that I don't feel I can make her happy? I tell her the other girl is the main reason. She gets upset, and tells me I should just be with her. I told her I do not like that reaction, and I do not need her advice. This could be the end. I am a little scared to call her.

8:01 p.m.: After watching porn for much of my life, I've gotten a false sense of the average penis size. I've come to the conclusion that my entertainment tool is larger than average. And I am pretty good with my tongue. I think that helps.

8:09 p.m.: I just want to chill in bed for a whole day with a beautiful woman. Maybe have sex like four times. I just told Monique that I want to sleep with an Asian and an Indian before I settle down.

10:12 p.m.: To my credit, I have been nothing but honest with the women in my life. Nevertheless, I believe I have hurt them unintentionally. In a year I will be engaged, and in a decade married with five kids, biological and adopted. I just don't know who I will be with.

10:56 p.m.: In the end it is going to be Monique or Jennifer, unless someone comes through and blows me away (figuratively and literally). Joking. I think I'm close to making a choice. I think within the next two weeks.

2

soloing

I AM MY OWN SOUL MATE

I'm single because I was born that way.

—Mae West

Seems a bit odd to become someone's other half, no? All the *communicating* and *processing,* not to mention the untethered agony of relationship books like this one. Why bother when you can simply meet all your needs yourself, and dip in for a bit of sex when time permits?

The two diarists ahead have no intention of ever entering a traditional sexual and romantic relationship, nor can they fathom why on earth their friends voluntarily cleave themselves to partners, potentially forever. They are soloists, meeting their own emotional, sexual, and financial needs through a mix of friends, family, and self-dependency.

Before this book, I published a British collection of diaries that included a genial, outspoken soloist known as The Porn-Loving Longtime Bachelor Who's Just Fine Alone, Thank You. He didn't find a partner to be a necessity, or even a frill, and was flummoxed as to why his friends were always pushing him toward *relationships,* with all their bells and whistles of cohabitation and wedding rings. "I suspect my friends desperately want me to say, 'I'm in a new relationship!'" he wrote. "People tell me I am nice, and so I should be in one." Pause for a moment. Imagine telling your best friend that he is so nice, but his abs are lacking. Or he is so nice, but his car is shabby. Exactly.

Soloism is a perspective that is rarely presented. When was the last time you saw a TV show about a happily asexual man, or a confirmed single-by-choice woman? In our culture, soloists are assumed to be seeking a fulltime mate—even the words "bachelor" or "single" imply their correlates, marriage and coupledom—despite the enormous evidence that they're not: 31.7 million Americans live alone, making up 27 percent of all households, according to 2009 Census figures. I assure you that 27 percent of all households are not in a frantic search to find an immediate cohabitating partner. The reality is that most diarists go through long stretches as soloists between relationships, and that at various points in their lives, many diarists *prefer* to be solo.

A Brief History of Soloism

Soloism was once considered the ideal state, by none other than Jesus. He valued his peers who devoted constant loyalty to God, and found that kids and spouses were time-consuming. Paul concurred, declaring that diaper changes distract men from the pious goal of serving the Lord (I'm paraphrasing here).[1] The New Testament is notably ambivalent toward marriage and family. The young Church eventually flipped its thinking when it realized that it had attracted a scraggly, impoverished bunch, rather than the aristocratic congregation of money and power it needed. So the Church began tapping into the social power of wealthy families, and encouraging childbearing. A few centuries later, Martin Luther declared celibacy to be unbiblical and not natural (note: it's quite biblical and perfectly natural); then Jane Austen wrote those oft-quoted words, "It is a truth universally acknowledged that a single man in possession of a good fortune must be in want of a wife." And ever since, flying solo has been considered a somewhat unnatural state. By the 19th century, Henry David Thoreau was justifying himself: "I never found a companion that was so companionable as solitude." Which is all to say that soloism, depending on where you are in time and place, can be the epitome of either social perfection or failure.

Today, soloism is perceived on the failure end of the spectrum, and what shines through in this chapter, more than the particulars of the diarists' lives, is the social pressure around them to become part of a pair. The Grandmother of Five, in her eighties, opens her diary discussing her hairdresser and daughter-in-law's encouragements to date. Her happy existence is an uphill battle against the assumption that she'd be happier sharing home, finances, and time with a man. It is no mystery why: nearly every commercial on television features some form of coupledom, either implied or visible; and though *Sex and the City* made the self-sufficient, stiletto-wearing model of singleness acceptable, the entire show revolved around getting unsingle. These diarists each live amid a wind tunnel of otherwise likeable, intelligent people who approach the diarists' solo status as a pesky setback to be overcome.

Much of the not-so-subtle disapproval that soloists feel—and in turn inflict on themselves—is, I suspect, because in America, singleness is quite new: Among people born in the 1930s, 96 percent married, and the handful who didn't were likely to live in family homes, rarely spending substantial time alone. Today, with microwaves and packaged food and small apartments and Internet shopping, living alone is the most common household style. Cultural mores just haven't quite caught up enough for people to be supportive of a friend meeting her own needs just fine. While I was writing this book, a slew of articles about the comedian Betty White appeared, all asking her whether she dates. I am here to tell you that if Betty White, in her late eighties, wanted another husband, Betty White would have another husband. The question is not, "Are you dating anyone?" but "How are you?" And if you really want to know, "What kind of soloist are you?"

In *Thinking Sex*, Gayle Rubin theorizes that society encourages lifestyles that it considers "good" and "normal," and marginalizes the others. Many solo diarists internalize culture's view of them, constantly second-guessing themselves, and questioning their value as people, their attractiveness, and their direction in life. The diarists in other chapters never do this—The Self-Employed Family Man or

The Outdoorsy Guy are in "approved" lifestyles of parenthood and dating and don't once give their lifestyles a critical thought. The diarists ahead are so woven into a culture that encourages relationships that they still think about themselves in terms of not being partnered. As The Bachelor put it, "Would laundry be any more bearable if I had someone to talk to and occasionally cuddle?" he asked. "No. Boring tasks are boring tasks, and drawing someone else into them is just that."

Soloists are not loners, nor lonely. The most curmudgeonly diarist in the book, The Grandmother Who is Perfectly Happy Alone, is in constant contact with her family, as well as a dozen coworkers. Soloists are simply choosing to fulfill their cravings for connection and meaning and dialogue outside of traditional relationship structures. Their diaries pull back the curtain on the endless diversity of lifestyles that people build to fulfill their priorities—like our next diarist, a grandmother who is quite content taking her morning coffee with a side of solitude. And you're blocking her view.

The Pleasantly Caustic Grandmother of Five Who Is Perfectly Happy Alone, Thank You Very Much

80, San Francisco, California

SUNDAY

11:33 a.m.: Had my hair done this morning. It looks good. There are two people in my life who say, "Nancy, you should date." My daughter-in-law—who is lucky I'm still talking to her—and my hairdresser. To me, it's too much work. I'm a different generation. The women stay home and take care of family and the man. Heck no. If a man asked me for a cup of coffee, I'd say, "Well, there's the kitchen."

12:00 p.m.: My situation is simple: no male involvement, and don't want any. I exist, take care of myself, and volunteer at a center for the indigent. My relationships are with my children and the people I volunteer for.

1:28 p.m.: Just looking out the window. Sunday is a day of mental and physical rest. I live in a big complex, and can see a gas station and a California employment office, which is about the ugliest part of the city. But the apartment is perfect for me.

2:30 p.m.: My son is visiting. My marriage brought me four wonderful children, who are my best friends. What could be better? We talk about a heartbreaking client I have been volunteering with, and about my late husband. He was reliable. He let me stay home and raise four kids. There was always a lot of food on the table, and I still had some money to fool around with.

7:00 p.m.: I will read and watch *Law & Order* for the next couple of hours.

MONDAY

8:00 a.m.: Turn on the news right away, to see what's going on in the world. As you can see, my life is always the same, week to week. It's alright. I find it comforting.

9:30 a.m.: Cooking a pot of oatmeal. Want comfort and love? Cook yourself some oatmeal. Whole oats, of course. Not the instant kind. Dreams are made of this stuff.

11:54 a.m.: Just did some exciting tasks. Ironing and cleaning the kitchen. Too excited—I have to sit down.

12:00 p.m.: I'm getting ready to go volunteer. Come to San Francisco and you can see my new handbag. You should see what I've done to my wardrobe since my husband died. He was a bit of a cheapskate.

5:20 p.m.: Had a good day today with volunteering. Actually helped some people. God, where are these people's families? I can't understand.

6:00 p.m.: Just got groceries. I stopped cooking when my husband died. Now I buy any prepared food I can find: chicken pot pies, V8 juice, yogurt. No more zucchini and rhubarb rotting in the fridge.

6:05 p.m.: We were married 40 years. When we married, I knew I could count on there always being money in the bank, and he'd probably never cheat on me, which I'm sure he never did. It ended with his death fifteen years ago. He quit smoking, but too late. Emphysema takes a long time. Eleven years. He believed in being as bitchy as possible. Some people approach death in a different way. We got through it.

6:10 p.m.: I retired and moved here two years later. I thought it would take me two years to get over his death. It took five. Which surprised me. I honestly don't know why. In some ways we were friends, and there was a small amount of passion—but he didn't have the same ideas toward women that I did. He thought, "You're the wife, you do the kitchen work and take care of the kids, and I'm a god."

6:12 p.m.: I guess 40 years is a long time to be with somebody. Some widows get remarried within a couple years, but me, no. I wasn't crying every day—it was like a veil. I was trying to look through a veil, and it took that long for the veil to lift. And now I'm off and flying.

9:34 p.m.: Watching *Law & Order.* I look at the men and think they're attractive. I like masculinity. But I guess I don't have any sex drive. And masturbation—no, no, I don't think I ever have. And now I'm 80 years old, for Christ's sake.

TUESDAY

10:00 a.m.: About to call one of my sons. I talk to them all once a week.

10:34 a.m.: This one and his brother are unmarried. I work at not intruding. I find it interesting how they interact with the people in their lives. It's the way I learn about them.

10:36 a.m.: My husband and I were definitely in love at the beginning. I didn't marry for convenience—I was supporting myself with secretarial work. I was tall and blond with big aids [breasts]. Our sex life was pretty good. Very enjoyable; nothing elaborate. I was a virgin when I married, at 24, and we had sex twice a week for the whole 40 years.

4:22 p.m.: Good day today. Client had a good day today. I so enjoy volunteering. Sun is shining, blue sky finally, everyone is happy.

6:30 p.m.: Eating a chicken pot pie. Enjoying it. At my age, I exist on memories. I envision a boyfriend sitting across from me, but that's just it—I find men are too immature and time-consuming for the rewards.

7:30 p.m.: Watching the news. It's a routine, but it's comforting. I enjoy it. I figure in these last years of my life I should learn as much as I can. I get publications from universities. I find I can only absorb what I want to know from books in the silence of being alone. So, no loneliness. I am trying to be a better person because I want to be.

9:30 p.m.: Going to bed. People ask a lot whether I'm lonely. Jesus always had people complaining to him, saying they didn't have this or that. And he said, "I am enough for you." And when I feel like maybe I should be more social, I think of that, and then that feeling disappears. So that's basically it. ✳✳✳

Sex and the Soloist

It is eye-opening to explore how sex fits into life through the diary of someone who lives in its absence. Most soloists are particularly skilled at discerning the correlation between sex and relationships—that sex is just one need that relationships can fulfill. The Asexual Filmmaker is no exception, and he is in the thick of unhappily parsing where he fits in the world, aware that he is far outside the paradigm of boy-meets-girl sexual relationships. And yet he still looks at his body through the prism of mainstream sexuality, and thus considers it a failure, which it is not at all. He blames his unhappiness on his sexuality, but he is actually a case study in poor social networks—his loneliness is a stark contrast to The Grandmother's.

Roughly 10 million Americans are asexual, meaning a life not *driven* by sexuality, but not necessarily devoid of arousal. The Filmmaker is very much motivated by the other two of the brain's three love systems (romantic love and long-term connection), and looks to fulfill them—just not through lust. All three diarists in this chapter are celibate, along with 1 in 5 in the general adult population (it's a U-shaped curve, with the youngest and oldest most likely to keep their trousers on). Celibacy has many faces, including The Single Virgin Obsessed with Sex who might not make it through the week without, as the kids say, swiping out her V-card.

It is striking that all three diarists in this chapter lack a model for their lifestyles, to the point that both The Asexual Filmmaker and The Single Virgin are unclear where to look for relationship partners.

Neither has friends or role models like them. "There's this idea that we *have* to be sexual," says sexologist Dr. Betty Dodson. "I gotta tell you, partners come and go. And everyone has a right to stop sex, or take a vacation, or not do it at all. Just enjoy your own body." Get a massage, take care of yourself, she says. Get your needs met in whatever way works for you.

The Asexual Filmmaker Who Doesn't Know He's Asexual

26, Denver, Colorado

SATURDAY

12:30 p.m.: Wake up. Making your own hours is like making your own muffins. They always come out weird compared to the kind the company makes. It's snowing remarkably hard today.

3:00 p.m.: Start work. I miss having an office. Of course, when I was on the job, all I dreamed about was staying home and making my own films. Today I'm fishing through public domain films, marking down timestamps for little bits I want to use.

7:00 p.m.: Take my roomie out for burgers. He's feeling down about having to move back in with his parents at the end of the month. I feel for the guy. I'm moving into my own place, first time in my entire life that I'll live alone. I haven't told anybody this and doubt I will, but I wonder if the loneliness will bother me. I'm kind of scared.

10:30 p.m.: Goddamn, it's still snowing. I'll have a cigarette on the porch. Roomie is singing along to the *Cheers* theme song in his room.

2:00 a.m.: Finally feeling tired. I attempt masturbation, but tonight everything's even more broken than usual. I can't even keep a woman's voice in my head long enough to feel anything—I start hearing song lyrics or my own breathing.

2:04 a.m.: I won't dance around it anymore: I'm a virgin, and in the last 10 years, I've had fewer erections than I did in the first two weeks of puberty. I'm not a sexual being. I need intimacy far more than I need some organ to spout goo.

SUNDAY

1:15 p.m.: Dreamed last night about fixing up an old house for my parents. There's nothing I want more in life than to buy my parents a house and support them so they never have to work or apply for food stamps again.

1:20 p.m.: The only reason I know I'm straight is the occasional half erections that slip past when a great pair of tits catches the whole mess by surprise. I've never gotten one of those for a guy, so I guess that's as definitive as I'm gonna get.

1:37 p.m. Taking out the trash. There's a young woman who lives down the hall from me, maybe 22 years old. Short, with red hair that bobs up and down, and green eyes that sparkle like copper fire. A tattoo of something with rings on her shoulder. World-class breasts, which have caused half of the aforementioned half erections.

1:40 p.m.: I try to start a conversation about the snow, which given the weather, isn't even a stretch. She answers monosyllabically.

1:48 p.m.: Big day of writing ahead. I don't want to do any of it, but oh, well.

6:12 p.m.: My laptop has died, again. Such fun, this electronic age.

7:46 p.m.: I just read this sentence on the Internet: "Don't be ashamed to talk about masturbation. Everybody does it or thinks about it." I embody that "or." I may not jack off very often, but I still fantasize. I fantasize about holding a girl and telling her about my day, about the warmth of a shoulder through sweater yarn, or the sensation of a held hand. Those are my dreams. That's what I want.

9:00 p.m.: It looks like the laptop is gone for good this time, which is fantastic since I just spent two days getting software on it and working on data that's now lost.

9:02 p.m.: I have never had a functional relationship with a functional woman. I'd describe myself not as "single" but as Separated. Martian. I've also never really enjoyed dating. It's amazing how little drive you have to go out and meet people when you're not looking for sex.

11:55 p.m.: Order a pizza and do a little painting. Life's not so bad.

MONDAY

1:25 p.m.: Wake up when the phone starts ringing. Talk to my dad for a bit, he asks rather incredulously, "I didn't wake you up, did I?"

"No, of course not." The rest of the conversation is sort of a blur. I think I fell asleep again.

4:00 p.m.: Working. I remember a girl I had a crush on in the 7th grade. Everyone assumed we were boyfriend and girlfriend. I asked her one day. "Would it be so bad if we were?" She answered, "Yes. It would be bad." And I remember that hurting a lot. After a moment she added, "But that was a great way to ask."

6:30 p.m.: Visiting my parents' house for dinner. A family friend just reenacted my previous relationship like so: She held up one finger, saying "You." She held up another, saying "bullet," and then shot one at the other for a narrow miss.

6:32 p.m.: You probably want more. She was a girl from Alaska. Eating disorder, lack of confidence, rape victim. She also had, buried under all of that, a great sense of humor and creativity and genuine goodness. We lived together for six months after knowing each other for three years. We never had sex. My lack of interest and her body issues kept either of us from suggesting it, but we cuddled a lot.

10:59 p.m.: Just back. I've only ever brought one girlfriend home, the Yukon Special mentioned earlier. When she moved out, my mother just shrugged and told me to try again.

3:22 a.m.: Waiting for my sheets to dry so I can hit the hay. Just thinking that I can't remember the last time somebody sought out my company specifically. This week has been particularly hard for my internal monologue.

TUESDAY

1:00 p.m.: I awoke from a dream to find myself fully erect for the first time in months. Not just a feeble attempt, but a full-on raging salute that, with malfunctioning equipment like mine, actually hurts a little. In the dream, I was floating at sea in a barrel. Dazzling against the sun was a beautiful senorita pirouetting atop a big glass egg. She was gorgeous, jet black hair and a strong but sleek physique and ample bosom. She smiled at me and danced away on her rolling egg as it floated away.

1:05 p.m.: I take advantage of the erection, first thinking of the senorita, but finding more solace in the redhead neighbor. I had forgotten how good sleep is after an orgasm.

2:00 p.m.: Still sleeping.

3:00 p.m.: It's raining outside. The trees are really beautiful when they're wet.

3:30 p.m.: Now it's snowing. Heavily. HEAVILY. Wow.

5:00 p.m.: Out to get a burrito, and I try something new: I look every person I meet squarely in the eye and try to think about how they're beautiful. I know, saccharine, right? I don't mean in the whole "everybody's beautiful in their own way" sense, but I mean looking at their faces aesthetically. Checking what color their eyes are, how they wear their hair, and so forth. The people respond by being oddly warm to me. Perhaps I'm on to something.

5:15 p.m.: I'm sure this sounds facetious, but I'm fascinated by the idea of giving a woman sexual pleasure. I have little hope for my own gratification, but driving someone else to it. . . that's got a ring to it.

6:35 a.m.: Just finished a *ton* of work. Sleep.

6:36 a.m.: I love being a night owl. The rest of the world runs on such a tight spring.

6:38 a.m.: You want to know what little naughty fantasy nibbles at me? I'll tell you: Conversation. A real, honest-to-God conversation with a woman. Not that goofy early part where you blabber compliments (though that stage has its charms), but that comfortable stage you get to if you do it right. The ongoing dialogue. Engaging with each other. Communicating without fear of judgment or estrangement. Sex is just a component of a more complex state of being with someone. I know it's there. I want the big picture.

· · · · · · · · · · · · · · · · · **Diary Insight** · · · · · · · · · · · · · · · ·

The filmmaker and the single virgin are young (26 and 23). Throughout the diaries, younger soloists tend to be more contented with their solo status, and it's because they treat solo as their native state. Because it is. They have spent 90 percent of their life in solo, and thus meet all of their own needs without much thought. A Saturday night alone is not a crisis for a 23-year-old. It's just Saturday. It's an attitude that older soloists can learn from.

· ·

The Single Virgin Obsessed with Sex

23, Dayton, Ohio

WEDNESDAY

4:17 p.m.: Just woke up. Last night I stayed up until 5:30 a.m. in the morning texting a married Albanian man. My best friend has been trying to hook us up for years, but we live in different cities and have never met. We'll meet at her wedding in two months. I feel conflicted: How much does "married" count if it's a green card marriage?

4:18 p.m.: I'm trying to stay a virgin until I get married, for many reasons. But I feel a long way off from marriage, and a short way off from having sex. Frustrated.

8:02 p.m.: Just got back from buying my maid-of-honor dress. Everyone around me getting married and having sex isn't helping.

9:20 p.m.: I can't stop listening to "Your Face" by The Frames. Not my usual kind of music, but right now I'm missing kissing. It's been 51 days, and that was a less-than-satisfying kiss with a good friend.

11:31 p.m.: Just done working out. I'm trying to get back into shape—I figure, if I let myself get out of shape now, who's going to want to have sex with me at 30?

11:35 p.m.: Reading back over these entries, I'm surprised by how much I think about sex. I want my thoughts to be more about *filio* [friendship] and *agape* [spiritual] love, and less on *eros*. I'm disappointed in myself.

3:44 a.m.: Married Albanian calls. I ask if he is single, to test him on whether he'll lie. He tells me about his marriage and the reasons behind it. My heart is pounding. I wonder if they have sex or sleep in the same bed. I wonder if God would consider it adultery if I kissed him at my best friend's wedding?

5:45 a.m.: Another late night, texting my Albanian. I text because I can say what I'm really feeling without having to sweat out any awkward, real-time reactions. After I said good night, I masturbated thinking about him. It was good. I masturbate almost daily. I use my fingers, outside my underwear. It's weird, but it's what works for me.

THURSDAY

11:04 a.m.: My religious beliefs are the reason I'm a desperate virgin at 23, and the reason why I'm very picky. I'm a Christian, and it's biblical, though often that's not what stops me from having sex. I hate children, and an accidental child would kill me. I also feel like I've waited this long, and I'd feel gypped if I gave it to someone who didn't deserve it. At this point, the only person I want to be that open with is whomever I marry.

11:06 a.m.: I'm grateful that I was surrounded by people with the same beliefs growing up, or I think I'd be a whore now.

12:00 p.m.: I see my ex tagged in a picture with a beautiful European girl in his arms on Facebook. When I was working in Europe as an au pair earlier this year, he became my lover (sans sex). Things ended two months ago when I cut my stay short to move to Dayton, where my old friend from college needed a roommate. My stomach feels like it's in an elevator.

3:39 p.m.: Just got back from my parttime tutoring job. I'm really encouraged by my student, and it's nice to have some social interaction.

8:06 p.m.: Trying on bathing suits at Target while on the phone with my little sister, who's younger and married. She tells me she once stole a dress from Target. She always makes me laugh.

10:00 p.m.: I've been so conflicted over whether to have sex. I've always thought that I would remain a virgin until I got married. I feel like I'm slowly being brainwashed by those around me into thinking it's not that big a deal, and that everybody does it. All I think about is sex; it's consuming my thoughts and I hate it. I feel like I'm going to explode.

12:54 a.m.: Just watched a documentary on sex, and it was fascinating. I should've been a sex researcher, like I always wanted to be in college, but I just couldn't imagine telling my parents. They would be mortified. They are extremely conservative Christians, and I don't tell them anything about my relationships, let alone anything sexual. They probably still think I've never kissed anyone.

FRIDAY

1:00 p.m.: Woke up thinking about how lost I feel. I've been out of school nearly two years now, and I'm nearly directionless. All I want is to be back in school.

6:25 p.m.: Just home from tutoring. He's 18, does math at a 6th grade level and has a baby on the way. He is nice, but he's ruining his life. Babies ruin everything.

8:15 p.m.: Watching fascinating documentary with my roommate about women trying to make it in the porn business.

10:32 p.m.: Just off the phone with Albanian. We had a 2.5 hour conversation about friendship, demons, movies, intelligence, cultures, money, respect. I want to kiss him, and I keep fantasizing about pulling him into my hotel room after my friend's wedding.

10:39 p.m.: My Albanian is passing 18 miles north of me. He's a truck driver. I want to go on an impromptu road trip. Ignore urge.

11:11 p.m.: Drinking; not tired yet, even though I have to get up at 5:00 a.m. tomorrow for my other parttime job. I'm making a wish for 11:11 p.m.: I want to meet my Albanian! *Shhhhhh*, or it won't come true!

11:55 p.m.: Sleep. I miss sleeping intertwined with someone.

SATURDAY

5:25 a.m.: Dreamed that I was the star of an Albanian porn movie, and I was trying to memorize my lines. I still remember the lines.

1:47 p.m.: My ex-boyfriend from college called me at work, and it was good to talk to him. I think we were too passionate for each other; we were like an explosion together. He was talking about the only girl he's dated since me. I can't get over this ache when I hear of old flames moving on, yet I'm enjoying having moved on myself. I'm such a hypocrite.

2:51 p.m.: Ex-boyfriend just emailed asking if I'll meet up over spring break. I want to. I want to kiss him again. We had such great chemistry. Why am I thinking this? I have no feelings for him, and I have someone else I'm interested in. One guy is never enough.

11:45 p.m.: Reading a book that my European lover gave me as a going-away gift. He wrote a note in the back: "I hope that you had a good time. For my part, I had a great time in your company. Goodbye, pretty woman." I don't feel like I'll be done with him until I finish the book. Reading quickly.

3:56 a.m.: Phone with my Albanian.

SUNDAY

12:54 p.m.: Just waking up after an exhausting weekend. I wonder if the Albanian and I will keep up this pace for two months, until we meet. I wonder whether we're good for each other, or am I fooling myself?

1:00 p.m.: I need more guy interaction. I know very few people here.

7:07 p.m.: Just got off work and off the phone with my best friend. Planning weddings are such a hassle. She's usually so calm. I'm never having a wedding.

8:00 p.m.: The Albanian told me to check out composer Goran Bregovic—he knows I like Gypsy music. One of my New Year's resolutions is to kiss a foreigner, and I will try my hardest to do so. I think I'll marry one someday.

PART TWO

partnered

a brief
intermission

YOUR EDITOR'S SEX DIARIES EPIPHANY

In my first weeks editing sex diaries, at the time for a magazine, my editor asked me to include each diarist's relationship status. The choices were: *single, in a relationship, married,* or *divorced.*

Now, the only rule of thriving as a writer is to simply *do what your editor asks.* Pointing out a beloved editor's logical flaws is the strategic equivalent of informing your mother that her parenting style lacked *pep.* There will be conversations to which you're not invited, silence, and then the budding reality that no checks will be arriving anytime soon. And so I kept to myself the minor detail that half of the diarists I commissioned did not fit into any of the given categories.

And so each Sunday night in my Manhattan studio apartment, I played a baffling game of *Categorize the Diarist.* Take The Eligible Guy. I called him to ask his relationship status. He replied in terms of the woman he sees most seriously: "I just call her 'someone I hang out with sometimes, and sleep with on occasion.'"

What?

"Well, once in a while, I am still sleeping with other girls—and it's not, really, like, 80 other girls, but, you know, it's not really just dating her." Pause. "*She* might say we're dating."

My editor: "In a relationship. Definitely."

You see my challenge.

This was my first realization that when people use relationship terms like "dating" or "single," they're envisioning the way *they* dated or were single. A "single" diarist could mean anything: celibate and happy, or promiscuous and playing the field, or divorced and dating someone seriously. It's their definition. Which is how I learned that all of society is batting around broad, meaningless terms about mating, with no connection to the realities I was reading in the diaries.

This, of course, was confusing for me. Because the diaries are exclusively about those realities, in all their stark, sexy detail. Many diarists, like The Eligible Guy, were enjoying an entire reality that slipped right between the accepted categories of relationships. I considered using other terms, but they weren't helpful. Facebook shares my pain. Their millions of users choose from one of 11 relationship statuses: *it's complicated, in a relationship, engaged, married, in a civil union, in a domestic partnership, in an open relationship;* or *single, divorced, separated, widowed.* Note that many of these are overlapping conditions. And that "divorced" and "separated" essentially describe a past relationship, not the present. And that none describes The Eligible Guy.

At first I assumed that my weekly troubles defining diarists' relationships was a simple flaw of vocabulary. Vocabulary tends to convey its historical past—in this case, viewing relationships through either legal status (married, separated, single, bachelor, husband/wife) or sexual ties (celibate, monogamous, polyamorous*). Of the pantheon of imprecise ways to describe a modern human, citing their sexual and legal status ranks high. Example: "He's a 40-something bachelor." The sentence could mean anything. It's so loaded with connotation that it's funny.

A few dozen diarists later, it dawned on me that that none of these words describe how people actually *relate* to their partners. In fact, all the diarists were chronically vague on this point. It was a sort of black

---

*Polyamory: seeking multiple, simultaneous love relationships, with the consent of all involved.

box. When asked about their relationships, diarists standardly gave a four to six sentence answer, and even then, just described their history. It was like no one had ever asked them before. They are much more descriptive in how they described their relationships with friends: a "work friend" or "best friend from high school" or "shopping friend" or "sports bud." But lovers? A "husband" is just "husband," a term that doesn't at all indicate whether it's a passionate love affair, or a marriage of communicative practicality. What needs are these two people meeting for each other? Who knows? There is no nod to the connection itself. Which is baffling.

And it wasn't just diarists. I spent more than a few days poking around libraries, and found myself surrounded by books telling me how to find and maintain the communicative, sex-filled "relationship" of my dreams. But not one book actually defined what that relationship *is*. Which is the equivalent of a restaurant menu that only offers FOOD, or a Realtor selling HOUSES. I was reading diarists' experiences from the inside of their relationships, and was stuck using terms that vaguely explain behavior from the outside.

It was The Trader Who Will Fly for Sex who made my brain blow a fuse. He was a Wall Street banker who, from the outside, appeared to be a squeaky-clean, hard-working guy. And every few weeks he called in sick on Friday and flew to another city for a sex date that he had prearranged online, often with a biracial couple, often filmed for posterity. (My editor: "Awesome, definitely.") I deemed him "single," solely by a process of eliminating *married, in a relationship,* and *divorced.*

By this point, *Categorize the Diarist* involved tequila. My fun, sexy editing job was taking over my intellectual life.

This would all have been an editorial chuckle, the sort of topic neurotic writers dissect over beers in Brooklyn, were it not for the fact that vocabulary represents how we conceptualize things. And I had read enough diaries to know that many of our misunderstandings of relationships are set in motion by our black-and-white vocabulary: you are single *or* in a relationship. Married *or* single. Monogamous *or* polyamorous. Celibate *or* sexually active. These terms are not, actually, binaries—as proven by roughly half of the diarists whose bedroom behavior fell into the large sea of space between terms. Language shapes ideas; vocabulary controls the conversation; and ours leads us to utterly incorrect assumptions about what goes on behind the closed doors of others.

Fast forward three years and 1,400 diaries. In 2010, I compiled three books of diaries for the U.K., Italy, and America. For this book, I initially grouped all of the "married" couples together into a chapter—which was a train wreck. The following diarists in this collection are "married":

- The Sexy Stay-at-Home Mother of Three
- The Very Busy Gay Dad Platonically Married to His Kid's Mother
- The Retiree Who Loves His Second Wife More Than Sex

Aside from cohabitation—and keep in mind that mole rats cohabitate, too—these diarists have *nothing* in common. Nothing. Comparing "married" to "married" is sort of like juxtaposing the oeuvres of Ayn Rand and Danielle Steel. Intellectually questionable. And all kinds of wrong.

And all kinds of damaging. As I spent my nights poring over the words of diarists, I found a common refrain: Many worried that they were doing it *wrong*, not having as much sex as they should, not finding a new partner as fast as they should, not feeling as happy as they should. (Use of the word "should" in the diaries is always a red herring that diarists are comparing themselves to mythical ideals.) And the underlying source of their worry? Comparison. You'll see it throughout the diaries: The Stepmom in a Hot Long-Term Relationship quickly compares herself to a less-sexually-active married friend; The Obedient Fundamentalist Military Wife compares her sex frequency to that of her highly sexual best friend. Their minds naturally compare "married" to "married" and "single" to "single."

The effect is destructive. Every Sunday, I read married parents beating themselves up for only having sex once a month, despite building wonderful partnerships around family and *never* prioritizing sex. Single diarists looked wistfully at happily married friends, despite limiting their searches to tall men of rare ethnicity with soul mate compatibility. And many felt guilty. Really guilty.

As I neared my 1,500th diary, what I had initially assumed to be a cloying weakness of vocabulary revealed itself to be a much broader problem: I was privy to bedrooms around the world, and could see that many diarists did not have the context or vocabulary to define their own relationships. Instead, they settled for a kind of vagueness that not only blinded them to fairly evaluating their own relationships, but became impairing when they evaluated themselves in comparison to others.

And the reality? Most diarists were, for the most part, in relationships that were absolutely typical for *their* needs and/or *their* type of relationship; and more importantly, most diarists were living precisely the existences expected based on the priorities they'd laid out. Which they would see if they judged and compared their relationships and priorities on their own terms.

So. Let's fix all this, shall we?

The diaries capture how relationships are experienced, from the individual's point of view. So I reframed my perspective on relationships to match. Because if I have learned one thing from 1,500 diaries, it is this: We are all individuals running around, trying to get our emotional and sexual and logistical needs met. And some of us will do that in long-term monogamous relationships; others swear by singlehood and a vibrator; some opt for a phalanx of friends and a lover or two, or vice versa; a few stick to decades of serene celibacy. Many slide in and out of all four, and at various points, state that they're utterly committed to their current fad. All of these are fine decisions. So let's talk about them clearly, in terms of how diarists are relating to others.

When I read each diary, I begin by asking a simple question:

What is the main motivation holding this diarist in this relationship scenario?

I call this the SDP Test. Whether a diarist is a celibate hermit or a free-loving parent, the answer quickly unveils *why* that diarist is connecting or disconnecting in that way, by highlighting which needs are most important to the diarist—his or her priorities. For example, The Kink-Lifestyle Dad is married because he adores his wife—and his marriage facilitates his widely ranging need for sexual exploration. The

Photographer is single because she craves an intellectual/sexual soul mate and hasn't yet found one. If the answer isn't clear, sometimes I ask, *What is the gravitational force that's motivating him or her?*

One Sunday night, I stayed up all night applying this question to every single diary in my database. Which is how I discovered the thirteen priorities that drive diarists toward others over and over again. Yes, there are hundreds of smaller needs that keep diarists in or out of relationships (think "we have a lot of shared friends" and "I can keep our country club membership"), but each diarist points to two or three of these as his or her priorities:

The 13 Relationship Priorities
- Sexual exploration and fulfillment
- Parenthood and family building
- Financial security and support
- Division of labor (income, medical, parenting, etc.)
- Lifestyle and status attainment
- Intellectual or spiritual soul mate connection
- Kink or alternative lifestyle exploration
- Romance and passion
- Religious partnership
- Daily companionship and hobbies
- Creative communion
- Professional partnership
- Security of a life partner

Now, yes, of course, many diarists desire most of these things. But we are talking about priorities. A diarist desiring good sex is not the same thing as a diarist *prioritizing* fantastic sex as an ongoing, major personal and relationship focus (sex parties, workshops, etc.). Similarly, many diarists desire children. But having a child with a beloved spouse is not the same thing as a diarist prioritizing a plan to marry the perfect parent, build a house for seven, and fill it with adopted children.

It is important to note that no diarist has all—or even close to all—of their needs met by one person. And that many diarists, at various points, meet many of their needs alone or platonically.

Thinking in terms of priorities is exceedingly useful, because it not only creates a language with which to talk about how diarists are actually *relating* to others, but gives a sense of why. Let's take the common, bewildering scenario of the miserable diarist whose life appears absolutely perfect: she's gorgeous, has a great job, an attractive lover, and a spectacular house. And yet she's miserable. Why? Because none of her prioritized needs is getting met.

When the SDP Test is applied to the hundreds of diarists in committed relationships, it gives a quick sense of *what type of connection* any existing relationship is, by foregrounding the content of the relationship. A pattern arises. The diarists fall into three types of partnerships, dictated by the couple's shared priorities. I've summarized the defining features of each partnership here:

What Kind of Relationship Is It?

Lovers

Lover relationships are defined by a very deep mental, emotional and/or physical connection, which they enjoy exploring in all its forms. Lovers strive for immediacy and honesty with their partner *right now*, and if that disappears, they often break up. The purpose of the relationship *is* the connection, and their diaries are filled with activities to nurture it, like long processing conversations (often prescheduled), sexual exploration time, or creative endeavors. They receive most of their deep emotional support from each other. Lovers tend to live in the now, and are finely attuned to their partners, growing upset if their partner seems distracted or unpresent.

Relationship Priorities (2–3, not all)
- ✓ Sexual exploration and fulfillment
- ✓ Intellectual or spiritual soul mate connection
- ✓ Kink or alternative lifestyle exploration
- ✓ Romance and passion
- ✓ Creative communion

Partners

Partners build intimacy through shared daily activities and hobbies, and by serving each other—one or both enjoy taking care of the other and being useful, perhaps serving meals or managing medical care. Their diaries are filled with small gestures like calling during the day, or greeting each other at the door, and these gestures are how they express affection. Partners are true companions, and fundamentally enjoy having a partner-in-crime with whom to share life's details. They tend to be focused a week or month ahead: For example, they know that they're going camping next weekend, and want to plan the menu and driving route. There is no achievement aim of the relationship. Often married, these diarists will divorce over inattention or infidelity. They are "life partners" in every sense of the phrase.

Relationship Priorities (2–3)
- ✓ Security of a life partner
- ✓ Religious partnership
- ✓ Daily companionship and hobbies
- ✓ Long-term familiarity and habit

Aspirers

Aspirers are allies in every way: deep friends, bonded by tangible, shared goal(s) that are best attained in partnership. Goals might include family (facilitating a stay-at-home parent), career (a political couple), finances (prioritizing one or both spouses' incomes to reach financial status) or sex (high-octane encounters). Aspirers approach the world as a united front, and differ from Partners in that their unions center around spoken or unspoken achievements that they are attaining, which they will often quantify (i.e., "three kids, $100,000 per year, and sex twice a week"). Most commonly, they are parents with clear financial and/or sexual expectations. Aspirers often maintain strong and deep emotional connections with best friends, who they lean on for emotional support. These diarists tend to think in the future, and have tangible long-term vision and aspirations. If one partner's goals shift, the relationship is threatened.

Relationship Priorities (2–3)

✓ Financial security
✓ Professional partnership
✓ Lifestyle and status attainment
✓ Parenthood and family
✓ Division of labor (income, medical care, etc.)

You'll note that these are the priorities of the *relationship*, not the individual—it's quite possible to be financially driven at work, and not at all within the relationship. And of course, all three types produce couples that are great friends, with the capacity for great sex; some diarists' relationships shift from one type to another over time. I've added the priority "long-term familiarity and habit," because I've found that once diarists' relationships have passed the 7- to 10-year mark, a diarist's longstanding trust and comfort becomes as strong a reason as any for staying put. As one wife put it, "Gene is like my arm."

But how can relationships possibly follow such an overtly logical system, you ask? What about *love*? Passion? The heady state of attraction? Even those in the throes of love have priorities. For some diarists, a spouse with a high-earning job and membership at the polo club is the definition of passion (Aspirer); others are attracted to a life of passion and adventure (Lover).

Sometimes asking the converse question makes it easy to identify which type a diarist is in: *Which priority, if removed, would cause this relationship to crumble?* Envision a tower of Jenga blocks—which block would most definitely make the tower collapse? If a diarist quitting his high-paying job would jeopardize his marriage, he's likely in a Aspirer relationship; if a diarist's fading from constant conversation or sex would mean Splitsville, she's likely in a Lover relationship; if a diarist's decision to leave the church would cause anguish, then he is likely in a Partner relationship. Note that these exact same decisions would likely not threaten the other two types.

Discussing diarists' relationships from the priorities perspective is edifying. Instead of struggling to compare "married" versus "married," it becomes easy to evaluate a relationship on its own terms, opening

the floodgates to see the pros and cons of each, and look at how diarists are successfully (and not so successfully) getting their needs met,
and why. As you'll see in the next chapter, each relationship type leads
to a completely different life.

The priorities perspective also makes it easier to comprehend diarists with lifestyles very different from your own. Take the diary of a
suburban religious mother struggling to understand her grown daughter's marriage to a cash-strapped artist. "Can't she find an employed,
Christian soul mate?" she wrote one night. She is assuming that *her*
definition of a relationship is universal, and that *her* prioritized needs
were the same as her daughter's. They're not. Her daughter is in a
Lover relationship, and the mother in a Partner. And if the daughter
could sit her mother down and describe her marriage in terms of
needs, her mother could certainly wrap her head around it. She
wouldn't approve, but that's a different story.

Like any other conceptual map, the three relationship types are one
way of classifying reality. It is not a dogma. There are other maps,
including an entire self-help oeuvre devoted to compatibility—exploring why certain personalities and biochemical makeups click. (Helen
Fisher's *Why Him, Why Her* is recommended.) This is not a replace-
ment for those theories, but a follow-up: lust evolved to encourage a
wide range of potential sexual encounters; love evolved to encourage
resource expenditures toward one person; long-term attachment
evolved to enable parents to tolerate each other long enough to surpass
toddlerhood. As you'll see in the coming chapters, once a diarist has
firmly chosen a long-term partner, much of her day-to-day future is
shaped by the relationship's priorities.

3

dating

IT'S SIMPLE: I LIKE YOU, YOU LIKE ME.

It is not enough to conquer; one must know how
to seduce.

—Voltaire

Reading the five diaries in this chapter is like entering a pink haze—
the diarists send their partners gooey text messages and emails all day,
can't keep their hands off each other, and generally ooze with warm-
fuzzy feeling. Yes, they're all high on love, and you can get a contact
buzz through the page.

A bit of context on the powerful impulses governing these diarists'
brains: All five are what you might call biochemically in love, featuring
brains that provide a dopamine boost each time they see their partner.
The newly in love can spend as much as 85 percent of their time thinking about their love, says biological anthropologist Helen Fisher. It is
constantly on the back burner, sitting there right behind every thought.
(Remember this detail the next time you see, say, a head of state fall in
love.) "These brain systems are very primitive, and tend to overtake the
rest of the mind," says Fisher. "The brain's reward center is activated
when you're madly in love." This dopamine system kick wears off after
18–30 months, which is why many diarists spontaneously begin

questioning their relationships around the 2-year mark, and can't quite put their finger on what has changed. Something big has changed: They're no longer addicted to each other.[1] But in the meantime, the brain chemistry helps. A lot. "When you are madly in love, it is an obsession," says Fisher. "A good obsession when it's going well."

It's going well. Four of the diarists ahead are not yet cohabitating, and without daily household interactions, it's easy to see how the priorities of each relationship—the *content* of each type of relationship and the *way* they interact—shapes three very different, distinct life trajectories. If you take one point from this book, make it this: The type of relationship a diarist chooses dictates much of the details of their daily existences, from sex to daily interactions, best friends to financial stability. Yes, their whole lives. And as you will see in this chapter, organized by relationship type, it's rather predictable. With each diary, ask yourself: What would this relationship be like 5 or 10 years down the line?

Partners

Let's begin with Partners. It's safe to say that Partners are *the marrying kind.* They are all raring to go down the aisle. As The Lovestruck College Kid writes, "It is ridiculous to say this so early, and possibly a jinx, but I think marriage is a good possibility after we graduate." He's 20. He's been dating his girlfriend for 12 weeks. His marriage schedule is slovenly compared to The Blissfully Boring Soon-To-Be-Wife Waitress, who was engaged two months into her relationship. Throughout the book, you'll see that The Lovestruck College Kid is the *only* Partner not yet married or engaged.

Matrimony dovetails well with Partner relationships because it supports the exact same priorities as the relationship. For The Lovestruck College Kid, legally binding himself to his girlfriend would allow him more companionship, long-term security, and constant daily support—the same three needs his relationship meets in spades. Partners also generally respond well to structure, and you'll see him implement it throughout his life, including (adorable) bedroom rules in the name of gender equality.

The way these two diarists interact with their partners is also quite specific: proximity. "We hang out in the bedroom on our laptops," writes The Blissfully Boring Soon-to-be-Wife Waitress. "I search for jobs, and he reads manga. It's so easy for us to just sit right next to each other." Direct interaction isn't usually the point—her fiancé visits her at work, and talks to others at the bar while she tidies silverware. The Lovestruck College Kid describes a similar 24-hour connection to his girlfriend through text message and Skype, often leaving her up on the screen. These diarists build intimacy through parallel experiences, affirming their relationships by their very presences. When these diarists do talk to their partner, it's usually a low-emotion chit-chat, updating each other on what's happened. This is markedly different from the Lover and Aspirer diaries you'll read ahead, particularly Lovers, who purposefully push each other's emotional and intellectual boundaries. Partner diarists are companions, present in each other's lives in every sense of the word.

Both diarists prize treating their partners well, which they do through a dozen small formal gestures throughout the day, such as serving a partner coffee or waving goodbye in the window. These gestures often become rituals. "We always greet each other at the door if we can," says The Waitress, and "we end with a goodnight kiss, as always." These are two tiny events that she fills with significance; their absence would signal serious relationship strain. We begin on a sunny morning in Massachusetts.

The Lovestruck College Kid Discovering Sex, Love, and Magnum Condoms

20, Lowell, Massachusetts

FRIDAY

8:40 a.m.: Just woke up, and basically the first thing I do every morning is text my girlfriend good morning. We typically text all throughout the day.

9:31 a.m.: I'm home for the summer and just Skyped with GF for about 30 minutes. We talk basically whenever we can. I think that everything she does is adorable. Even when we don't have anything to talk about, we still talk, or just goof off in some way. I love her.

9:32 a.m.: We have been dating for over three months. It worries me that we have to be long distance for the next year because of her traveling abroad, then my graduating. So two years, actually.

12:57 p.m.: I went to the gym for a few hours today, which I am trying to do on a pretty regular basis. I have been self-conscious about how skinny and nonmuscular I am, because I want to look good for my girlfriend. She is really gorgeous, and I have always felt bad that I am not the "manly man" that you would expect to be with a girl like her. I know she doesn't care, but it's still something I think about a lot.

1:02 p.m.: Missed call and text from my girlfriend. She does not get upset when that happens, but I still feel a little guilty about it. I want to always be able to be there when she wants to talk.

10:54 p.m.: So this entire day, I have texted with GF at least a few times every hour. It's just what we do.

10:57 p.m.: Experimenting. Sometimes I have problems getting an erection with the condom on. It takes an embarrassingly long time. I have spent a lot of time online researching this, and see that it's common, but it is still pretty embarrassing. Just had particularly pleasing results. The problem was that the condoms were uncomfortably small. It is far easier to keep an erection with a Magnum condom. The Magnum condom fits on much better, doesn't fall off, and doesn't restrict blood flow. Talk about a self-esteem boost.

11:00 p.m.: My GF has told me I am big before, but I assumed she was trying to make me feel good.

11:44 p.m.: Bedtime for me! Just called GF to say good night. When we are at school, she usually sleeps with me. I miss being naked in bed with her, just cuddling and falling asleep.

11:48 p.m.: It may sound like I am totally whipped by my girlfriend. It is kind of true. But the thing is, I kind of love that. I think she is amazing, and should be treated like a princess. I am not exactly a prince charming, but I try as hard as I can every day to be a perfect boyfriend because I love her. She knows that, and she likes that.

SATURDAY

8:33 a.m.: Just woke up, and am off on a family weekend, which will be super super annoying. But I know I will be texting GF a lot. She makes my family bearable.

8:38 a.m.: I haven't really masturbated since I started dating my girlfriend. We started more heavily fooling around (hand jobs, blow-jobs) about three weeks into the relationship, and then about three weeks later we had sex for the first time. She was pretty shy about it because she was a virgin, which was fine with me. Then we were having sex once or twice a day, and I never had much of a need for masturbating. Now it has been four days since we have had sex. I am OK for now.

9:27 a.m.: I really like my sister's boyfriend. He treats her so well, and she seems really happy.

8:59 p.m.: Family event. All the parents keeps asking about significant others. My parents met in college. I try to tell my family as little as possible about my private life. For example, the first time my mom met my girlfriend, she said, "She reminds me of a mix between your last two girlfriends." This made me uncomfortable.

9:02 p.m.: My girlfriend is way prettier than my cousins' girlfriends, which makes me feel super cool. They were always the strong manly guys. I was always the loser. I win.

9:51 p.m.: So I have a tendency to talk in a baby voice, especially with GF. People have made fun of me. My sister told me she does the same thing. So do both of my parents. We just realized that it is because our parents do it.

10:08 p.m.: Tonight I have been lying in bed and I have started to worry that she won't want to stay in a long-distant relationship. It will basically be two years. I love her so much.

SUNDAY

11:00 a.m.: Hiding from my grandmother's birthday, so I'll tell you about us. We met at school two years ago, in the drama department. I was dating another girl, which was a bit of a train wreck. It ended very poorly, with her telling me that "she never really liked me that much in the first place." I was in tears. But it was my fault for not seeing the patterns of her standing me up and treating me badly.

11:05 a.m.: I spent a year trying to get my girlfriend to like me. When I finally got the courage to ask her out, she said no, then didn't talk to me for a month. Then we got cast playing romantic leads. For months she was leading me on, and I confronted her about it, and told her I didn't want to talk to her for a while. Somehow the next day, we hooked up a party, and went on a date that went . . . nowhere. Then we talked every day as friends over holiday break, and afterward she admitted she always had feelings for me, but was scared to admit it because she had never been in a serious relationship. When I changed my relationship status to "In a relationship," I literally got thirty responses from my friends saying they were happy for me.

11:45 a.m.: Fun Fact: My girlfriend shares the same name as my ten-year-old pet goldfish. I would like to think that this is a coincidence.

7:34 p.m.: I just arrived home. It was painful without cell or Internet all day.

7:37 p.m.: At school a lot of people are into just hooking up at parties. I can't do that. I am very bad at hooking up for a night. I am a long-term relationship person. When I was single, I was pretty unhappy. I really hate being alone. I just get sad. Generally girls do not find me attractive. I tend to be "the friend." But not now.

10:10 p.m.: Thinking about sex. I always feel a little bad that our foreplay basically happens the exact same way every time. But it's OK because we vary up sex. We joke that because we're both inexperienced, we're in sex training.

10:14 p.m.: Usually sex starts with us just talking, and then we start to make out. We have a rule that we have to be wearing the same amount of clothes. So if I take off my shirt, she must take off her shirt. It's all just to be fair. I start to kiss her neck, then her nipples. Then either I go down on her or she will go down on me. At some point before sex we both have gone down on each other. Again, we are all about equality. We still need to use a decent amount of lube because fitting into her is still a little hard because she is still very tight down there. Eventually I get her going, usually in missionary. Sex lasts between 5 minutes and 1.5 hours. The 1.5 hour day—that was just a miracle. I just like to do whatever she sounds to be enjoying the most. I can tell by her breathing what she likes. Once I am in the game, I do pretty good work. Once I am done, I get up and take the condom off, and then we cuddle for a while. I really like to cuddle.

MONDAY

1:31 p.m.: So GF and I Skyped for three hours. We started talking about who in school we think is going to get married and when. It was odd because clearly on both of our minds was, "What do we think is going to happen with us?" Neither of us said anything, because it would have been weird, but I know I was thinking it, and I bet she was, too.

2:56 p.m.: It is nice to know that we both want the same things in life. Our dream is to live in New York, working in theater, and have a family. It is ridiculous to say this so early, and possibly a jinx, but I think marriage is a good possibility after we graduate. For that to happen though, we need to stick through the long distance for a full two years. I think we can handle it. I want that. I want to be with her forever.

2:00 p.m.: We're texting. Back when we weren't "in a relationship" yet, texting was even more important. You use texting for basically all forms of communication with somebody that you are interested in. It's how you flirt. If you text too much, you seem too needy. Not enough, they think you are ignoring them.

3:14 p.m.: So I was really nervous before me and my GF had sex. It had been a really long time. About 1.5 years. So it was basically like losing my virginity again. I had issues with the condom, and I was really nervous because I really love her and did not want to be terrible. I had trouble keeping an erection. It was kind of a mess. However, when we tried again the next day, all was well.

3:20 p.m.: Here is a funny thing. When we started dating, I would ask if she felt ready, and we finally had sex one night. And from then on she became a SEX MANIAC. She is all about having sex all the time. I have no problem with this. But I just find it funny that she was a virgin one day, and then once she had sex once, she never wanted to stop.

7:00 p.m.: Back from gym. Two ground rules that we made for sex: no threesomes and no anal sex. We both think of sex as something special, and wouldn't enjoy it if someone else were in the room. My body is only mine and hers. Her body is only hers and mine. And as far as anal sex, we both think it's weird and scary. We have just started to explore sex in new, more risky places. Once we did it in a practice room at school, and once in somebody else's room when they were away. We are still exploring new things, and new places we can go. We take sex seriously, but we love to have fun doing it.

10:13 p.m.: GF and I Skyped for another three hours tonight. It was nice that we got to talk so much today. I really do miss her, though.

The Blissfully Boring Soon-to-be-Wife Waitress

25, Des Moines, Iowa

FRIDAY

4:48 a.m.: Wake up and let the dogs out. I always have problems sleeping after my fiancé gets up for work.

8:00 a.m.: Getting ready for my annual gynecological exam—those are always awkward. Nothing like some complete stranger looking somewhere that you only let one other person go.

10:00 a.m.: He's home for lunch. We hang out in the bedroom on our laptops. I search for jobs, since I'm losing mine at the end of the month, and he reads manga. It's so easy for us to just sit right next to each other. He's perfect for me and I'm perfect for him.

1:00 p.m.: Waiting at the front window for him to get home from work. He is getting off early so we can go get our engagement photos taken. We greet each other at the door if we can.

1:30 p.m.: "Getting ready for photos" turned into making out, which turned into sex. Every once in a while he'll come up with some new position he wants to try, which he did today. I'm perfectly happy with the usual two—him on top or me on top. I guess I feel like any other position makes it less special, like the action no longer means we love each other, and it's just a physical thing. But I do it all for him because I love him and it makes him happy.

2:00 p.m.: Brief discussion about our honeymoon schedule.

3:00 p.m.: Just barely made it to interview a photographer on time. He's using the photo session as an excuse to keep kissing me as much as he can.

4:00 p.m.: He decides to play video games rather than come watch *Star Trek* with me.

4:15 p.m.: He's making a pizza sub and asks if I want one, too. Granted, he has to ask me for instructions on how to make it, but it's cute. He brings the pizza subs into the bedroom and watches *Star Trek* with me, even though he doesn't like it.

6:00 p.m.: Every Friday during Lent, his mom puts on a fish fry for the Knights of Columbus. I go with them even though I'm not Catholic. We support each other's religions.

7:47 p.m.: Sat and talked with his mom for an hour while his dad disappeared. They only live a mile away, so we like to ride our bikes or walk our dogs to his parents' house. We have dinner there once a week. We talked about everything from careers to parenting (which included a really awkward comment about me using birth control). We have only had a couple of these talks, but they are getting easier.

9:00 p.m.: Movie, bed. We are way too young to be this tired and boring on a Friday night.

10:30 p.m.: I know he's trying to fall asleep to be up at 6:00 a.m. for work, and yet I keep wanting to have a conversation, since we're not really gonna see each other tomorrow.

SATURDAY

7:00 a.m.: He always kisses me before leaving, but sometimes I'm so exhausted that I don't feel it. Usually, we walk each other to the door.

9:15 a.m.: Just finished straightening the kitchen and sorting the laundry. I always said my husband would share the housework 50/50. I probably do about 80 percent, plus lawnmower maintenance (he hates it). But I'm used to doing all the work after taking care of my mom and grandma, and I'm older. If I ask for help, he does it.

9:18 a.m.: We've been together two years now. We started hanging out and then making out and then going out, and when I decided I couldn't live without him, I officially broke up with my high school sweetheart, who I'd been on-and-off with for five years. Then two months later he asked me to marry him.

10:00 a.m.: Just booked our wedding photographer!

1:00 p.m.: He just left to go back to work after eating lunch. It's amazing how something as simple as suggesting I make him some macaroni and cheese for lunch can make his eyes light up. Otherwise he just eats pizza and quesadillas.

4:45 p.m.: Sometimes when I leave for work when he's not here, I leave him little love notes just to make him smile, like "Love you forever" on a hot pink Post-it note on the front door. He kept it. We're pretty sappy like that.

6:00 p.m.: Saturday is the loneliest day of the week. He works all day, then I wait tables at 5. Thank God his schedule is changing and I will spend Saturdays with him.

10:00 p.m.: He came to see me at work. Right now he's having a couple of drinks with the parents of one of the kids he coaches. I love when he introduces me—especially when they tell him that he has such a beautiful fiancée. Face it: I'm marrying a blond, blue-eyed, captain of the high school sports team. And he's marrying a size six, long-haired athlete too.

11:00 p.m.: He's sitting with me as I roll silverware with the manager. We all talk sports. I'm really glad that he isn't jealous and doesn't mind that I have male friends. He trusts me 100 percent.

12:00 a.m.: He just left. The girls at work always say, "He's so sweet! Does he have any friends?"

3:00 a.m.: It's so nice to finally crawl into bed and snuggle up next to him before going to sleep. My favorite part of the day.

SUNDAY

9:11 a.m.: I can never sleep well after such a busy night. He can tell I'm grumpy because I yell at the dogs. I swear to him that I'm not. I am.

10:00 a.m.: Time to leave for Aikido class together. We try not to partner with each other in class so we can concentrate more.

12:00 p.m.: After the first class, he thanked me for going with him and said all of his friends would have laughed at him. It was sad, and at the same time, I know that he believes I'm not just his future wife but also his best friend.

2:00 p.m.: Romantic comedy!

4:45 p.m.: He's getting ready to coach. He wears these tight Under Armour shorts underneath his soccer shorts and they show off his package. I made an "Oooooooh" face, and he playfully covered himself up and said, "What are you looking at?" "Just watchin' the show." "There'll be another one at 8:30," he said. Quick kiss and then out the door.

5:15 p.m.: I'm a little disappointed because Sundays tend to be our day together. It's not that big a deal though.

7:00 p.m.: Making dinner. It's strange how such a simple act can make all the difference in a relationship. Making dinner for him is like taking care of him. I feel guilty when I leave him to fend for himself.

9:00 p.m.: Sitting in the bedroom on our laptops. I'm writing, he is playing computer games. He's lying across the bed, I'm using him as a desk.

10:00 p.m.: Some nights all we need is a little bit of foreplay and some oral. For us, it's about the closeness, the intimacy, not the physical gratification.

10:45 p.m.: Lying in bed, talking about past relationships. We find ourselves jealous of our previous significant others only because the thought that anyone else might have our affections is irritating. A silly thing to think about because we can't change it, and we believe there will never be anyone else.

MONDAY

9:15 a.m.: Facebook. My ex has decided to enlist in the military, and updated his status to "in a relationship." I was always a little worried that he was so hung up on me that he'd never date anyone else. At the same time, I am a little sad that he enlisted. I wish he would come back. I still care about him, of course.

1:00 p.m.: At my other parttime job. A friend brought over her Chihuahua. I texted him that I want one. Response: "No. No. Bad." We already have four pets.

3:45 p.m.: Changing clothes. He's on his laptop not paying much attention. It's a little strange because usually when my top is off I have his full attention.

4:30 p.m.: I write out all the bills every month. He's never been shown how; I always watched my mom. But he just looked at the due date for one, and said he thought we needed to send it in today. I think he's learning.

6:55 p.m.: Text: "You're more beautiful than the first snow in quiet woods and nicer than the first sunny day of spring when the flowers are in full bloom. I love you."

8:00 p.m.: He's visiting me at the restaurant. I wasn't expecting him today. I tell him that he doesn't have to come see me every day, but he likes to.

10:00 p.m.: He gives me a much-needed neck massage before bed. I have such a great man, and know that all the other girls are jealous. We just fit together perfectly. It's like a Venn diagram that's all shared area.

10:30 p.m.: Finally climb into bed after my late dinner. He snuggles up next to me and tells me that he will always be here for me, and I tell him I know. We end with a goodnight kiss like always. In our private life, things are perfect. We just wish everything else would fall into place as easily. ***

Lovers

You're in for a treat. Lover diarists are endlessly entertaining, due to their penchant for ignoring all practicality in the name of love. The Marketing Guy Hosting His Long-Distance Boyfriend is a New Yorker about to move to the Deep South where he knows zero other people. The Madly-in-Love-17-Year-Old is mind-bogglingly unfazed by potential teen parenthood, noting that her boyfriend would have to "quit wrestling and kickboxing." These diarists would live in igloos if their partner suggested it.

Yet there is a rationale to their pink logic. These diarists, above all, prioritize the immediacy of their intellectual and physical connection, and will do whatever they need to do to nourish it. And so, in this chapter, the Lovers are happily setting themselves up to spend the next few years (if not decades) managing the life complications that may ensue. Practicality be damned.

These diarists are in the exact same stages of new love as the Partners, yet display a completely different way of interacting with their partners. The Madly-in-Love-17-Year-Old takes morning walks with her boyfriend, during which they talk about "all things philosophical." She prizes honesty at all times, at one point writing him "a nice letter about all my thoughts, rendering them naked to him." The Marketing Guy does the same, writing his boyfriend "a long email, which I then cut down to a few paragraphs telling him how awesome the weekend was and how much he means to me." Their relationships pivot around emotional honesty and immediate expressions of what they're feeling right now.

Note that none of these diarists even mention marriage. Throughout this book, few of the Lovers are married. It's because marriage doesn't support their goals. The concept of marriage is fundamentally based on staying together in the future, and Lover diarists live in the present. Lovers crave informal, constant connection *right now*, and if that involves nudity, even better. Planning a formal future ceremony doesn't support that goal; in fact, it's rather opposed to it. Compare this to The Boring Waitress, who is gleeful to book a wedding photographer. Lovers are not against marriage; it's just not a priority. They'd rather be in bed.

A new perspective on marriage emerges through the diaries: it's quite clear that marriage supports a specific set of relationship priorities, which apply to only half or so relationships (Partners and some Aspirers). Marriage is the equivalent of buying a house. Over 80 percent of the population does it at some point in their lives, often for smart reasons that support their life goals. But it wouldn't make sense to blindly encourage all Americans to go by a house. Which is exactly what we do as a society when we constantly inquire whether wedding bells are forthcoming.

We begin in Manhattan after an early morning workout.

The Marketing Guy Hosting His Hot Long-Distance Boyfriend for the Weekend

28, New York City

TUESDAY

8:05 a.m.: Lying in bed post-workout, trying to load gay porn. Internet is being stubbornly slow, so I tap into downloaded reserves. Agree to allow myself 15 minutes with a few Eastern European gods.

8:38 a.m.: Still going at it. Look at clock and tell myself I have *got* to get in the shower . . . right after these last two pool parties. Make an impromptu segue into a video that my long-distance boyfriend, Mark, made for me a few days ago, of him jerking off in the shower. Does the trick.

9:15 a.m.: Waiting for L Train, the bane of my existence. Make awkward eye contact with a semi-cute college boy. He's wearing a V-neck so low that you can almost see his happy trail. American Apparel must be stopped.

10:45 a.m.: At my marketing job, instant messaging with Mark. He's ten years my senior and lives in Alabama, which might as well be Afghanistan. I met him seven months ago at a bar when we were both traveling, and we subsequently started visiting each other every weekend. By the time I was permanently maxing out my MasterCard, I was in love. I never thought I'd ever do something like this, but he's all kinds of awesome and ultimately so worth it. He's coming to visit in four days. Cannot wait.

7:30 p.m.: Lying in bed jerking off with Mark over Skype. He tells me to spread my legs and finger myself. This sends him over the edge. I watch him explode onto his stomach and then I come all over my stomach and chest.

WEDNESDAY

7:45 a.m.: Watching a video of a twink in his boss's office getting fired for insubordination. "But I have car payments!" he pleads. The boss says the twink can keep his job only if the boss can "breed that hole." Twink's reply: "I'm usually straight but, my damn car payments . . ." The delivery of this last line cracks me up. I rewatch it again and again and make a mental note to show my roomie, hoping we can make "my damn car payments" into a thing.

7:50 a.m.: Realize I've been lying alone in bed naked cracking up to amateur porn for five solid minutes. Jesus.

1:45 p.m.: Mark is in a three-hour meeting. To help him get through it, he begs me to go into the bathroom in my office, take a picture of my flaccid penis, and send it to him. I reply "no chance in hell, mister."

1:55 p.m.: Walk past guys at the urinals, and enter the handicap stall of the bathroom. Try to wake my cock up so it's not *too* flaccid. I grab my balls, lift my package up, take out my BlackBerry, and snap a pic. But damn it's not on silent mode! The camera flash sound echoes throughout the tile bathroom. The dudes totally heard that.

1:59 p.m.: Wait patiently as the last dude finishes washing his hands and leaves before making my exit. Wonder if there are surveillance cameras in these bathrooms. That's illegal, right? Mark owes me a killer blowjob for this.

2:09 p.m.: Mark's texted response: "Mmmm." That's it? Notice he has refrained from using exclamation points in his texts and emails as of late. Think about bringing this up.

2:10 p.m.: Decide I need to dial down my internal crazy.

7:05 p.m.: En route home, I run into a 23-year-old restaurant manager that I was mildly obsessed with two years ago until he stopped calling me. He says he just moved in around the corner, and he'll hit me up on Facebook and we'll grab a drink. I've been a good boy for six months. Cannot screw up this relationship.

8:05 p.m.: Consoling roomie who is recovering from a breakup. (He found an active Manhunt.com account on his boyfriend's computer, and further proof of hardcore cheating in archived instant messenger chats.) We drink boxed wine and watch Glee.

11:03 p.m.: Restaurant manager boy instant messages me. Says his on-again-off-again boyfriend is out of town. I tell him I have a boyfriend of my own. He goes idle.

11:05 p.m.: Think about the night we drank Red Stripes and I gave him head. Immediately text Mark, tell him how lucky I am to have him.

THURSDAY

8:00 a.m.: Browsing videos of presumably real fraternity boys forcing their pledges to have sex. Guess I was in the wrong fraternity. The videos are ridiculous. But kinda hot.

3:00 p.m.: Mark sends really sweet texts that quickly devolve into dirty ones, including a picture of him standing in front of the mirror holding his porntastic, 9-inch penis. I start typing a text that says "your dick belongs in the Smithsonian," but decide it's too lame.

10:15 p.m.: At a gay bar in Chelsea wing-manning for roomie. I must be exuding some sort of relationship-induced confidence, because I keep getting the eye, way more than I ever do when single.

10:20 p.m.: A cute-enough Latino flirts with roomie. Says he's an actor. From Queens. Hello red flags.

11:00 p.m.: Roomie is making out with the actor. That didn't take long.

11:15 p.m.: Taking a piss in the bathroom. Eye-flirt with scruffy hipster. I am hopelessly turned on by arty, bespectacled hipsters.

12:30 a.m.: Stumble out of bar and drunk-dial Mark. Have exceedingly cutesy, lovey-dovey talk that I wouldn't dare repeat to anyone. He tells me not to jerk off that night or the next morning. He wants me fully loaded when he gets there. Gulp.

FRIDAY

8:00 a.m.: Back watching a video of a really cute young guy being forced to recite the alphabet as he blows his brother's beefy best friend. Weird.

8:10 a.m.: Notice I am out of lube. Remind myself to pick some up after work for the weekend. Mark will be here in mere hours!

12:30 p.m.: Lunch with friends at a Cuban joint. Tell the friends that I'm probably moving to the South later in the year. Friends ask if I'm on meth. Mark can't get out of his job contract, and my life is far more malleable.

1:30 p.m.: Mark tells me he's leaving for the airport soon. Penis twinges at the thought of impending sex.

3:30 p.m.: Brainstorming something special I can do once Mark arrives. He always goes all out when I come to his place. Blanking on ideas.

6:30 p.m.: At Rite Aid buying cigarettes and KY Warming Gel. Of course, there are two grandmas and a WASPy mom standing in line behind me. No, I don't have or want a goddamn club card, cashier lady. Just put the lube in the bag.

7:40 p.m.: Mark has landed in JFK. I sip on a Stella, cursing myself for not at least getting flowers or something. I scour the apartment but can't find so much as a candle. In roomie's room a piece of red ribbon catches my eye. Contemplate stripping naked and tying a little bow around my penis. Ridiculous. Wonder if it's cute-ridiculous or oh-my-God-we-are-breaking-up ridiculous.

8:15 p.m.: Lie naked on my bed trying to tie this stupid piece of ribbon around my junk. The air is cold and I'm nervous and my dick is stubbornly receding inside my body. The schizophrenic little bastard.

8:18 p.m.: He buzzes up. I can hear the elevator descending to the lobby.

8:19 p.m.: The ribbon is tied. Am I really doing this?

8:20 p.m.: I'm going for it.

8:23 p.m.: He enters out of breath and immediately cracks up at the sight of me. I sit there with a shit-eating grin and he picks me up and I wrap my legs around him and we kiss hard. I love how strong his upper body is and how he can pick me up so effortlessly (I'm over six feet, mind you). He carries me back to the bed and in what feels like seconds his clothes are off and he's fucking me.

8:30 p.m.: He clutches my hair as he comes inside me. I finish on his chest. We cannot stop kissing.

10:30 p.m.: At a late dinner with friends. He sends me a text: "I cannot wait to fuck you again."

12:35 p.m.: At a gay bar in Chelsea making out in the corner. A drag queen on a microphone makes fun of us. We are so *that* couple in the bar, but I don't really care.

2:00 a.m.: Back at my place having drunk sex. I reach my hand around and massage his balls as I ride him hard. He comes inside me again. I'm too drunk to cum, so we just pass out.

SATURDAY

9:30 a.m.: Mildly hung over, I awaken Mark orally and we soon segue into a 69. He starts to rim me. He doesn't like to be rimmed himself, so I focus my attention on his penis. He comes in my mouth. I've never been much of a swallower but with him I kinda love it.

1:30 p.m.: All-day brunchathon in Brooklyn. Buzzed on Bloody Marys, thinking about how we've been living in a perpetual honeymoon state of weekend visits and beach vacations all year. Start to fear what the unsexiness of daily life will do to us once I move in. I'm determined to make it work, in small part to prove all my friends who think it's a *bad idea wrong.*

4:25 p.m.: Day-drunk. Mark needs a nap. Roomie is home with the ex. I can hear them both crying in his room. Oh, lord.

6:45 p.m.: Mark bends me over in the shower. Officially sore now. Mark makes fun of me for being a "power bottom," a phrase that has always grossed me out. Tell him I've always been more of a top in experiences past, but he doesn't believe me. He's a total top, so it's not like I have much of a choice.

SUNDAY

9:45 a.m.: We wake up early and go for a run along the West Side highway. He breaks the news that he might have to work the week of my birthday. I'm bummed and a little confused as to why he waited until now to tell me, but I don't make too big a deal out of it. (I do, however, make a mental note to bring this up during our next fight.)

11:00 a.m.: We're all sweaty and he's sitting up in bed with his back against the wall and I'm riding him in a circular motion which he loves. I come all over him, and continue to ride him hard until he comes.

11:04 a.m.: On a post-orgasm high. I tell him he's the best sex I've ever had. His playful response: "Wish I could say the same." Paranoia ensues.

1:30 p.m.: At brunch. Getting really sad. He's leaving. Weekend flew by as usual. Trying not to come off too desperate and emotional, but I can't help it.

5:00 p.m.: Cuddling in bed. He has to pack soon. I'm teary-eyed. He says he wants to make love one more time. I tell him I might be too sore but he promises to go really slow.

5:03 p.m.: He puts me on my back and I wrap my legs around his lower back and grab his ass. Slow, tender sex ensues. He sucks on my tongue as he comes.

5:40 p.m.: And he's gone. I go cuddle with roomie. Big sigh.

MONDAY

8:00 a.m.: Skip morning fun and go workout. Not really horny given the weekend sex binge. Barely make it two miles on the elliptical. Ass is beyond sore.

11:20 a.m.: Write Mark a long email which I then cut down to a few short paragraphs telling him how awesome the weekend was and how much he means to me. I won't get a response for a while as he's on a long flight.

4:30 p.m.: Mark sends me a sweet response.

8:30 p.m.: On couch with roomie drinking more boxed wine, watching more Glee. Thirteen more days until I get to see my guy again.

The Madly-In-Love-17-Year-Old Who Might Be Pregnant

17, Southwest Houston, Texas

TUESDAY

6:49 a.m.: I had ten minutes to get ready. After Sam snuck out, I brushed my teeth to expel that lingering salty taste. He crawled through my window last night when my mom was working graveyard shift, as he occasionally does. She has gotten used to our relationship, but I don't think she'd approve of me sharing a sleeping bag with him.

9:00 a.m.: We've been together for 27 months. Our lives are intertwined and dipped in glue. Inseparable.

2:17 p.m.: Got busted for PDA in the hallway. It's always the same old grumpy lady who shoos us. Don't be jealous just because you've never had a hot guy fall in love with you.

4:06 p.m.: Still feeling that little tug in my stomach from Sam telling me that he found another girl "appealing." What is the logic in telling your girlfriend that? Anybody?

4:08 p.m.: By the way, she's blond and she and I are what I guess you can call . . . "friends."

6:06 p.m.: Walking home from school, bracing myself for my mom's sympathy-seeking while she complains about her boyfriend. And she has the nerve to tell me Sam and I aren't in love.

6:08 p.m.: After my mom found out that Sam maxed out my v-card [virginity], he's permanently on her naughty list. The woman's even cussed him out. Ah well, no worries.

7:00 p.m.: I'm so glad to be back in Houston. When I moved away to my dad's house for a year, all Sam and I had were phone calls. And cameras. It was really hard, but there's a strong connection. Nothing can break it.

8:19 p.m.: Big plans for tomorrow. I'm making breakfast for Sam and I can't decide between pancakes and eggs or pancakes and waffles. I love the feeling I get when Sam eats my food ravenously. It's so flattering.

WEDNESDAY

6:49 a.m.: So Sam didn't come over last night, but it's probably better, since he has a standardized test today. He wanted me to bike over to his house, but I was *way* too tired. I feel bad because he's usually the one to come over. But he understands.

12:43 p.m.: Today, this Hispanic guy with a greasy *fohawk* wouldn't stop hitting on me and checking me out in the hall. Since Sam and I have this agreement to tell each other this kind of stuff, I had to tell him. He got really jealous and cranky, but he's okay now. He knows it's not my fault.

2:46 p.m.: I can't wait for school to end. When it ends and we are standing in the crowd, it feels like we are the only two people in the hallway. The warmth of his chest is soothing and I love how he lowers his head to hear me better.

2:48 p.m.: We dated for four months before we first had (awkward and disturbingly quiet) sex. We have found a lot of privacy here and there while our parents are away or at work—though it doesn't look like we'll have any more this week.

5:59 p.m.: Bored. Groggy. Feeling fat. Sam said today that I was "too little," and I don't know how to interpret that. I know he likes that there's a significant weight difference between us. It's sexier. Even I prefer pornos where the girl is thin and the guy big. Don't know why.

9:36 p.m.: Still bored. Drinking some sort of chamomile tea. I have a poetry reading at school tomorrow and no idea what poem to read. I'll pull one off my closet wall. Can't wait to go on my morning walk tomorrow with Sam. It's our designated time to talk about anything philosophical that comes to mind.

10:00 p.m.: Sam's incredibly smart and he likes to debate with me, and he's very muscular. His eyes are amazingly cool. Ew, I'm so in love with that kid.

THURSDAY

6:51 a.m.: Sitting in my assigned seat at school, headphones firmly implanted in my ears. Now that I think about it, I haven't masturbated in a few weeks because Sam and I have been satisfying that hunger frequently. At random times, in random places.

10:21 a.m.: Still haven't started my period. Wondering. What would I do if I were pregnant? My mom would scalp me and Sam would quit wrestling and kickboxing. Not too worried, but a little nervous. I haven't told even my best friend.

3:00 p.m.: I'm a very jealous person, so when some chick comes up to me and says she saw my boyfriend get out of a car with a blond girl (the girl he likes)—I freak.

5:30 p.m.: We had a big fight. He was not planning on telling me.

5:41 p.m.: Fuck my life. I'm seriously contemplating one of those nice little morphine capsules hidden in my secret stash.

8:50 p.m.: Crying. Insecurity sucks. I have small boobs and a not-so-narrow waist. Pimples, frizzy hair. I don't get amazing grades and I'm not particularly good at anything. No job, no car.

FRIDAY

10:59 a.m.: Wrote a nice letter to Sam about all my thoughts, rendering them naked to him. The release was amazing. I feel like my honesty can only take our relationship further. Can't wait for fourth period to end, so I can read his response.

1:02 p.m.: Mood: apathetic. I just want the weekend to embrace me. Oh, the update on my period: nowhere in sight. Lovely.

3:30 p.m.: Oh, jeez, that fight was bad. No yelling, but I just felt altogether hopeless and worthless. I'm usually hesitant to complain about things that make me jealous, because I don't want to nag. I don't want to be one of those women who can't just let stuff go.

6:06 p.m.: After school I came home and ate 12 Oreos, 8 Nutter Butters, 1 bag of chips, 1 mango, crackers and cheese, 1 tortilla, 1/2 a Sonic foot-long Coney, and some tater tots. Did I mention I have kickboxing in an hour?

8:12 p.m.: I feel shitty.

SATURDAY

8:06 a.m.: I am a bit hoarse from last night's crying bout. I don't want to be too quick to forgive, as is often the case, but I kind of need to, since he's my ride to kickboxing. Not eating much.

12:45 p.m.: Skating alone. Oh, how I love the skating rink. Last night's zolpidem (a sleep pill) has me drowsy, but I plan on having plans tonight.

5:20 p.m.: Elated. Just adopted a pit bull with my mom! Her name is Gorgeous. She's so sweet. Somebody to give me unconditional love! I want to show her off to Sam, but I'm still wounded from last night.

7:06 p.m.: Gorgeous is so attached to my mom's boyfriend, and it has me jealous. He didn't even go to the shelter to adopt her. Grrr. I will officially introduce her to Sam tonight even though I smell like mud and wet dog.

10:42 p.m.: It's so messed up how Sam gets me horny right before he has to leave. We were sitting on the couch and he was rubbing my no-no triangle through my shorts. Is there a female equivalent to blue balls? I think so. But most of the attention was on my dog.

SUNDAY

9:20 a.m.: So lazy. I am still in my pajamas and Sam is out lifting weights. He's gotten pretty muscular since we started going out. I like his body. All I know is that I can't get fat because he's such a health nut.

1:09 p.m.: Please tell me I'm nauseated because of the shrimp. I feel sick and fat today and I want to see my boyfriend so that we can talk about what we'd do if I was prego. FYI, he kind of wants a baby.

3:00 p.m.: Biking to Target for a pregnancy test because my boyfriend was too horny to pull out. If I was pregnant it'd work out.

4:56 p.m.: I saw him talking to *her*, and got a bad taste in my mouth. Is it fair for me to be this jealous?

8:00 p.m.: Not pregnant. Sam said he was relieved, but disappointed. I was, too.

8:10 p.m.: We've talked about trying 69, but haven't had enough time. It sounds fun.

MONDAY

7:03 a.m.: I am feeling spectacular today. Sam and I met up this morning for our walk. He is the only one for me. I realized that I can't give up on our relationship every time we fight. My relationship is the most intense thing I've ever known, and sometimes it's unstable, but I like it.

11:05 a.m.: Super sleepy and hungry. Gonna get our salads and enjoy the fresh air and privacy of the outdoor picnic tables.

1:00 p.m.: Did I mention I'm feeling pretty content? Maybe it's because I started my period!!!

8:28 p.m.: Yum. Mint tea. No plans for tonight but to read *The Scarlet Letter* and text my baby. The drama is slowly dying down, thank God.

10:30 p.m.: Just got off the phone with Sam. We talked about joining a commune. I'm psyched. Major headache. Goodnight world, Mom, sis, Sam, Rosie (yeah, I renamed my dog). Goodnight diary. ✳✳✳

Aspirers

Make-up sex is the domain of Aspirers. They need it. Especially in the early phases of their relationships, which are often spent ironing out what the shared priorities of the relationship will be. Fights are common among Aspirers, because they are sometimes wildly different individuals who disagree on many points outside of their shared relationship goals. These are the couples you know where one is Republican and the other Democrat, or one a Type-A parent and the other a *laissez faire* farmer, and you can't figure out how, exactly, they're together. They're together because they want the same things—and have the same relationship goals. This is where the make up sex comes in. Aspirers constantly use sex as a tool to smooth over their many individual differences. This is unique to Aspirers—Lovers tend to see sex as a means of communication or path to spiritual enlightenment; Partners enjoy it, but deprioritize it. For The Finance Dad, sex is a high point in his life, but also more often than not serves the very practical purpose of paving an escape from a screaming match. They fight; sex ensues; they calmly go about the rest of their evening. The underlying problem is never resolved, but as long as their larger goals are aligned, it doesn't need to be.

The Finance Dad's relationship structure is typical Aspirer: he knows exactly which goals he'd like to achieve and maintain through his relationship (sexual fulfillment and financial sanity), and those two points form the core of their connection. They approach the world as two allies who will achieve their goals against all odds, and the world better look out. Aspirer diarists are the marrying kind when legal marriage supports the goals of the relationship—which, where children and finances are involved, it usually does.

Yes, dear reader, The Finance Dad is clearly on the narcissistic end of the spectrum, certainly not a trait shared by all Aspirers. Diaries like this one are, however, helpful in understanding the minds on Wall Street, most of who opt for Aspirer relationships.

The Finance Dad Marrying His Mistress, Whose Daughters Are Siding with Mom

44, New York City

MONDAY

10:40 p.m.: It's been a long week of parenting and working, and it's my last night at home before visiting my fiancée, Claire. Yay! I can't wait for my week with her.

11:56 p.m.: I just said good night to Claire on the phone, and my son is asleep, but I'm not ready for sleep myself. Decide to view a favorite starring Tia Ling, from the archives.

12:20 a.m.: I love watching girls climax! I wish I could be that helpless. Wonder if we'll get any bondage in this week. I've also been hinting that pegging is on the menu—I'm a virgin in that way.

TUESDAY

6:00 a.m.: Morning wood. I ignore it and get going. I am head over heels in love with Claire. Before I met her, I had a 17-year (or maybe a 44 year) dry spell, and I've been trying to make up for lost time with a willing partner. Unfortunately, she lives in another city with her child, while my kids are here.

6:30 a.m.: Touch up on man-scaping.

7:00 a.m.: I walk to the subway with my crabby teenager. I worry he's angry that I'm leaving tonight. I have alternating-week custody, and I can't do anything about it, so I keep silent.

8:30 a.m.: Status update call with my company's foreign office. I get distracted thinking about going down on Claire. The nice hard conference table would be perfect.

9:30 a.m.: Meeting finally ends. Place a wakeup call to Claire.

10:30 a.m.: Call ex-wife to coordinate children. Yuck.

3:57 p.m.: Watching the clock. I can't think straight. I'm ready to be in Claire's arms.

7:45 p.m.: Doze off on plane fantasizing about Claire taking advantage of me and straddling my face. Would love an extended scenario where I am her property.

9:20 p.m.: Hugging Claire at the airport is as sweet and powerful as the first time four years ago. I forget all my worries.

10:30 p.m.: Fairly heated discussion with Claire about dealing with the financial consequences of divorce. Not fun.

11:15 p.m.: We both catch up on email and work before bed.

12:15 a.m.: We go to bed. I try some foreplay, which makes Claire fidgety. She can't take it anymore and decides to tie me spread eagle to the bed. Victory! She's well-rested and in no particular hurry. After taking a few orgasms for herself, she finishes me off. The combination of time apart, bondage, and the build-up just blows my mind.

1:12 a.m.: Claire unties me, but she's not quite done. We try out a vibrating toy we've never used before–two silver bullets attached to a controller. It works.

1:20 a.m.: I'm the big spoon tonight. Life is great.

WEDNESDAY

9:10 a.m.: We go at it again, further exploring the new toy.

11:26 a.m.: In my marriage, there was no intimacy, emotional or physical. I had no idea what I was missing. We met in college, and I was far too inexperienced. The few times I tried adventures, it would wind up in tears. So very bad. I never cheated, except for one incident with a physically-satisfying lap dance with a stripper, with whom I felt an emotional connection. That was my warning sign that I ignored.

12:00 p.m.: Working. I am lucky, and can do my finance job on the road.

5:13 p.m.: Sex on the brain again. Starting to wonder if I'd be greedy enough to try for more sex later.

12:15 a.m.: Watch a couple of old episodes of *Sex and the City*. Naked. Amuse myself by rubbing up against Claire. She is receptive. We go to bed. A bit more rubbing and bingo!

2:00 a.m.: Despite our best efforts, I am unable to orgasm. Claire has had several. Masturbation, assisted by Claire, works. We spoon.

THURSDAY

6:30 a.m.: Morning wood. Roll over and go back to sleep.

10:30 a.m.: Claire is prancing around the house, first in nothing, then undies, then partially and then fully clothed. She looks amazing in every configuration. I love my life.

5:00 p.m.: Lawyer call. Legal wrangle with ex intensifies. She was shocked when I told her I was leaving, and we've been in protracted legal battles—she definitely wants to see me suffer. I am on edge for the rest of the day. Claire and I discuss my custody agreement for my children. We communicate poorly. Silent treatment ensues.

5:05 p.m.: My romantic advice: counseling. I wish I had put my ex-wife and I into counseling after the stripper incident. I've seen this pattern with some of my friends—men don't call for counseling when they should. By the time I was in love with Claire, I wasn't prepared to risk that relationship to handle my existing marriage appropriately. I also don't understand much of my twenties. Every time someone tells me that their spouse "wants the same things out of life" or "will be a great parent," I cringe. I was just on a train, and jumping off was too traumatic.

7:31 p.m.: I should say that Claire and I had an emotional affair, and things didn't become physical (although she was willing) until I decided I was ready to move on. I told her that I thought she might be the one I wanted to spend my life with. She was extricating herself from a marriage that was also deeply unsatisfying. We made quite a spectacle of ourselves on the street, making out during a blizzard. We finally got together for a weekend away. It was electric, emotionally and physically. I was afraid for a few days afterward that I was broken. A month later, we left our spouses. We've both been divorced for two years.

1:00 a.m.: Go to bed and have it out. Fight. I am getting chastised although I did nothing wrong! She's frustrated because my daughters don't spend as much time with me as they're supposed to, and if they're not going to, why am I in their city? I think she is just frustrated at our situation. I stick up for myself and feel completely alone.

1:15 a.m.: My situation is more difficult. My family is in a boys vs. girls situation. I did lot of stuff with my son that took me away from my wife and daughters. They made a "girls club" and my relationship with my daughters has suffered.

1:30 a.m.: Anger has dissipated, and, somehow, sex seems possible!

2:10 a.m.: Claire laments that she can never finish me with oral. I inform her that her prospects are better after a dry spell. She wants to try anyway. She ties up my arms and it seems like it should work. Then she gets turned on and has to bang me. She has two orgasms. Claire resumes oral, bangs me again, and eventually we both finish. I don't know why oral isn't enough by itself.

FRIDAY

9:25 a.m.: Crawl back in bed to wake up Claire. A brief-but-yummy cuddle.

10:50 a.m.: See what's new at Kink.com.

6:30 p.m.: Going to the climbing wall. We're talking about sex: our first times, and how teenage boys differ from teenage girls. All this bodes well for tonight.

7:00 p.m.: Claire is playing with me in the parking lot. We're not above vehicular sex, but this parking lot is too active.

10:00 p.m.: Get dinner and categorize all our female acquaintances as lipstick, wand, or sybian. Fun game.

1:00 a.m.: She's exhausted. So am I, although I'd still rather make love. No chance.

SATURDAY

9:30 a.m.: Wake up and start playing with Claire's body. Our no foreplay rule gets brought up and I tie up her hands. Claire can only tolerate manual or oral stimulation when she's thoroughly turned on—she finds penetration too intense. So we often start with penetration. It doesn't take—she's free again. We pull out all the toys we can find and everything is clicking.

9:40 a.m.: It's a great session. When she's going down on me, I have a lot more freedom to do whatever I want, namely go down on her.

11:00 a.m.: Fall back asleep.

11:30 p.m.: Try to interest Claire in sex. She laughs at me. It's too soon. Cuddle up and watch *Sex and the City* reruns.

SUNDAY

9:45 a.m.: Now I'm definitely interested in some action. But Claire's kid is coming over soon, and we have back-to-back activities until tonight. Frustrating.

4:40 p.m.: I'm done working, and we wind up alone, watching *Sex and the City*. We discuss the episodes. Talking about sex usually leads to sex. This time is no exception.

4:45 p.m.: Claire's kid stops by to pick up a gym pass. Major mood killer. Afterward, I persist. A role play. The scenario evolves to me providing Claire admittance to a secret society. Props: blindfold, ottoman, rope, vibrating bullets, glass dildo.

6:10 p.m.: Claire's kid returns with the gym pass. The bedroom is toy heaven. Super annoying.

MONDAY

8:05 a.m.: Check out what's new at a kinky online porn site. Consider masturbating, but decide to wait and see what the day brings after work.

6:00 p.m.: Claire comes home in a bad mood. This makes me very edgy.

11:30 p.m.: Claire tries oral on me again, and almost brings me to orgasm. However, Claire gets too turned on and we transition to sex in the spoon position. Fall asleep inside her.

4

committing

TOGETHER, FOREVER

> Love is an ideal thing, marriage a real thing. Confusion of the real with the ideal never goes unpunished.
>
> —Goethe

You might note that the diaries opening this chapter are chock full of sex. This is not a ploy to lure you onward (though I'd do it). It's because frequent sex is a hallmark of Lover relationships. In fact, the three Lovers ahead are so sensual that I was unable to find a diary without a sex act in the first entry. We all have our professional struggles.

The six diarists ahead are living the American dream, immersed in happy, long-term relationships, occasional grumblings about dishes notwithstanding. On the outside, they seem to be fairly interchangeable couples. Their diaries tell another story: three completely different realities. Different because what each relationship *consists* of is wildly different, beginning with basic spousal roles. To The Sexy Stay-At-Home Mom, a spouse is someone who appears for family breakfast and dinner, pays all the bills, and keeps her sexual fires lit. To The Lesbian Sex Educator, a spouse is a spiritual soul mate, and financial solvency and shared meals is less relevant. If you squint your mind's eye, you can see how, five or ten years ago, these relationships resembled the duos from the previous chapter.

The lives that flow from Lovers, Aspirers, and Partners differ so dramatically that you'll ask yourself, "Wait, how did I never see this before?" You didn't see it because you've never read their diaries. The *content* of a relationship is among the most secreted information in an adult's life, not necessarily shared with even a best friend. You have to read their diaries to find out.

Lovers: My Life Is Hot

Why so much sex among the Lovers? Because these diarists prize a constant, immediate (intellectual, emotional, spiritual) connection with their partner. And sex is an effective way to achieve that. These are not people who have sex for the sake of having sex. Instead, these diarists use sex as an exceedingly sensitive form of communication, with a quality of depth that you won't see in the other diaries. And the *role* that sex plays in these relationships is unique as well. While Partners and Aspirers frequently use sex as stress release, and find that a roll in the hay ameliorates all sorts of interpersonal sins, for these diarists, the sex is a continuation of the constant communication that they are always in, talking, touching, thinking, and chewing on ideas. Sex appears at all times of the day, as part of the normal flow.

Some background information: The average American has sex 62 times a year—or once a week, plus a couple of times on vacations.[1] That figure is heavily age-dependent, dropping by around 20 percent per decade, mostly due to health problems. Marrieds under age 30 have sex twice a week. When age is controlled for, sexual frequency is stable throughout long-term relationships—and Lovers are off the charts. The Lovers here have sex almost daily, and when they don't, they tend to do a lot of sensual touching, constantly feeding their connection through cuddle-and-conversation. You'll see that Lovers are also much more flexible in their definitions of what sex *is*. Since it is mostly a form of connecting, they are much more likely to engage in mutual masturbation, sexual touch, and other non-intercourse activities.

These diarists rarely mention shared daily tasks or finances, because it's not a core part of their relationship; their unions have not necessarily improved their socioeconomic outlook. (Compare this to the Partner and Aspirer couples in this chapter, *all* of whom involve one spouse largely supporting the other.) Of the three Lovers ahead, two manage their incomes separately; only The Lesbian Sexual Educator mixes money and love, and their business relationship is clearly secondary. This is not to say that these are not career-driven diarists—all are pursuing ambitious careers. Just not through their relationship. Instead, their partner is their best confidante on Earth.

Author Ayelet Waldman set off a firestorm in 2005 when she wrote in the *New York Times* that she loved her husband, the author Michael Chabon, more than her four children. She didn't garner any further peer support when she added that she suspected that she was the only mommy at Mommy and Me getting laid. Her article reads like a playbook to a Lover relationship, where the connection between the two adults is, above all, the goal, and everything else (children, money, etc.) comes second. Yes, these are the diarists that you might catch gazing into each other's eyes at the supermarket, in a way that would make many Partners or Aspirers feel uncomfortable.

The Upstanding Schoolteacher Dad Who Would Like Some Triple-X Time

32, Ouachita Parish, Louisiana

FRIDAY

8:00 a.m.: First morning of summer break, and my wife continues our tradition of a good morning blowjob and breakfast. With a start like this, the stack of grading is hardly daunting at all.

1:15 p.m.: Damn the French and their cinema. Watching a movie, and the last scene has me missing my wife's bottom, giving it a squeeze, but she's off shopping.

4:18 p.m.: In passing I touched her ass while she cooks. Such a lovely thing, a woman's ass. I reflect over the fine memories I have of my wife's ass.

6:00 p.m.: I doubt that I masturbate more than five times a year. Since January, however, that number has increased and I'd bet I've masturbated more in the last five months than in seven years of marriage. A couple of times I've done it in front of her. She masturbates fairly frequently herself and has throughout the marriage. It's helped me be more attentive to her when we do have sex. With three young kids and a newly pregnant wife, we've remarkably been able to give each other some enjoyment twice or thrice a week.

9:02 p.m.: An endless graduation ceremony has drained my libido. I rehash the horror to my wife as she bathes.

10:06 p.m.: Conflict. My wife volunteered me to babysit the difficult nephew, along with my kids, tomorrow while she and her sister attend a lingerie party. So no sex.

SATURDAY

7:00 a.m.: An early jump on the day precludes sex this morning.

7:11 a.m.: I am hopeful that a morning praising sexy underwear will get my wife in the mood to pull out some of the numbers I've gotten for her over the years.

10:44 a.m.: Looking at photography sites. I share a few sexy pictures with my wife. I debate sending along a picture of two fat people, he in jeans holding a sword, she clinging to his side absolutely naked. It's gross, but romantic. And—I suspect for them—totally hot. I describe it to her instead.

11:55 a.m.: Babysitting. I've gone from idle horny to full-on horny. My wife returns from the lingerie party soon.

8:23 p.m.: After a long day the kids are in the tub. Just another half hour and we can unwind. Having three kids has made sex almost strictly a post-bedtime activity. Sometimes we can sneak in an early morning session, but the risk is walk-ins. When it happens you slide into the most unassuming position and ask for a few minutes before getting breakfast.

8:38 p.m.: My wife, when tired or busy, is usually open to bump-on-a-log sex—she the log, I the bump—but I don't care for that. Which is not to say that I didn't accept on numerous occasions. Lazy sex made us both feel guilty, her for not being more into it, me for hassling her.

9:20 p.m.: Wife comes onto me while I'm brushing my teeth. Earlier in the year we talked through our expectations and desires. I thought that she was less interested in sex and she thought I was less desirous of her. We were trying to get pregnant and I was frustrated by the cursory nature of sex at that point. Over a couple of nights we hashed out the problem, a month back she conceived, and everything's been smooth.

9:50 p.m.: We talk in bed. We don't have sex every night. We do, however, talk every night in bed. I opted for the best-friend-and-lover amongst spousal types. I knew from an early age that I wanted someone coming from a different cultural direction. I wanted polyphony, panorama. The current formula for romantic success is craven for sameness. I wanted difference among shared beliefs and loves. I wanted to pull and be pulled, transformed into something new. That's what I got in my wife. We work together, we struggle, we come together. We have sex, both come, then go to sleep.

SUNDAY

7:38 a.m.: We have a fish fry today at noon, then kids' friends spending the night. I don't foresee much private time today.

8:27 a.m.: The boys are playing with a radio and have found Elvis. "I'm in love. I'm all shook up. UH HUH HUH." They think it's pretty comedic.

3:17 p.m.: To list some things about my wife that I like in no order: that she spends as much time on the aesthetic arrangements of her meals as she does on the taste. I love the way she dresses, which includes a style unlike any I've ever seen, and the physical act of clothing herself, how she peeks at her body in the mirror, like she is impressed, preening, and critical all at once. I love her slightly asymmetric teeth, which are far more interesting than dental Chiclets. I also love the way her eyes crinkle when she smiles, which is pretty conventional praise, I know.

3:19 p.m.: My wife is so much more different than any list of likes I would've made the week before I knew her. Before I favored more petite women, smaller breasts, athletic, sharp-tongued, and she's more curvaceous with bigger breasts. But she's transformed my desires.

Those little dinky girls look so insubstantial to me now. What I think is beautiful in other women is what I recognize from her in them. I like aspects in other women that I love in her.

5:07 p.m.: Listening to romantic songs. I'm constantly wanting her to dance for me. She's pretty cool toward the idea of me dancing for her.

7:16 p.m.: I unloaded, she reloaded, the dishwasher.

9:29 p.m.: I'm wondering if I'll get special treatment tonight. I've done some pretty selfless acts today.

10:34 p.m.: Wife and I talk in bed. She reminisced about the birth of our second son, whose birthday is tomorrow. She recalled having sex and waking up later thinking the flow back was her water breaking. I'm pretty sure this is her idea of sexy talk.

MONDAY

8:31 a.m.: After mowing the lawn and breakfast, I'm thinking of stealing away with the two-year-old while scads of five-year-olds go apeshit in the backyard. As I get older I'm less and less interested in other people's kids.

8:32 a.m.: Children are the ultimate extension of your penis.

11:00 a.m.: I've suggested creating a trove of all the sexual accoutrements I've purchased over the years, so that we can incorporate them a little easier. Out of sight, out of mind. I'll pull out the lacy gloves and thigh-high socks and waggle my eyebrows a little. She is self conscious about her body, but I've more than made it clear that her pregnant body is a fetish of mine.

2:04 p.m.: Starting to fear that I'll accidentally put one of these entries on Facebook.

2:44 p.m.: I just remembered the time I had sex with my wife out in her father's wheat fields. My birthday a couple of years ago.

6:41 p.m.: I think I'll be requesting head tonight if it isn't proffered.

6:42 p.m.: My wife is afraid that I prefer oral sex over other forms. I understand why, but the reasons are misleading. I do make more pleasure noises when receiving head, but because she's requested them as a sort of sonar. When performing sex I'm concentrating on a variety of things: how I'm feeling, how she's feeling, how long we've gone, how long we'll go. But when receiving head I'm just enjoying the moment, how it feels, how she looks giving it.

6:59 p.m.: I suppose all men think their wives are beautiful when going down on them. It surprised me how sexy it is. Especially since it's such a comedic-looking thing to do. And what's more ridiculous than the end of a blowjob? How we keep from laughing is beyond me. Actually, sometimes we don't keep from laughing.

7:04 p.m.: And ultimately this is why porn is such a goddamn bore. No comedy. This whole putting a bit of ourselves into a bit of someone else is weird.

10:11 p.m.: Heading to bed after a ridiculous movie. Pregnant wife is highly emotional and we're both tired.

11:30 p.m.: In bed we kiss briefly and talk while I manually stimulate her. Once she comes, she gives me head despite her oncoming cold. I'm a bit surprised by how into it she is. A long day succumbing to sickness doesn't normally lead to a good time in bed.

11:35 p.m.: For the record, I like giving head more than she likes receiving it. She says it's her chief fantasy, and she orgasms, but I offer four times before she'll accept it. I consider oral sex as a regular part of the meal and sometimes the main course.

TUESDAY

6:43 a.m.: What's the deal? I don't want to be awake right now. The wife is sick and I'm in the beginning stages.

8:08 a.m.: I don't want to go in to do that last bit of grading.

9:28 a.m.: I'm heading to the office and taking the two oldest with me. Wife is off shopping with the youngest. I gave her ass a squeeze before leaving. I've really turned into an ass man.

3:05 p.m.: I just read some Basho, the Japanese haiku poet, to my wife that held some innuendo. She's off her game, she didn't catch it.

3:12 p.m.: My wife was upset when she bent over in my presence and I didn't flick her skirt up. Sheesh, I'm off my game.

4:39 p.m.: I told my wife that I wish she were cooler sometimes, in the hip sense. She's quirky hip and her own person, which is attractive to me, but she isn't sunglasses cool. She took it the right way. I used to be cool. It's easier for guys to be cool. I had my own kind of cool. For girls they have to be more standard cool.

4:44 p.m.: For some time I've scoured eBay for a leather mini skirt. It'll be the post-pregnancy motivation for dropping the weight.

9:15 p.m.: The wife and I watch a movie featuring one of her crushes, Penelope Cruz. I drink tequila and rub her legs.

9:22 p.m.: Change the computer background to Cruz in red negligee. It tickles me to surprise her like that and I can't wait to see what she'll replace it with.

10:32 p.m.: Discuss the motivations for ejaculating on a woman's face. We draw no conclusions.

10:42 p.m.: We talk in bed about past romantic encounters, which, bless her, spawns a new romantic encounter.

· · · · · · · · · · · · · · · · · Diary Insight · · · · · · · · · · · · · · · ·

In this chapter of committed couples, diarists repeatedly use their fantasies as just that—imaginary tales that have nothing to do with their current partner. Both The Stepmom and The Female Minister fantasize of orgies and sex with women. In chapter 6, The Successful Consultant imagines her previous, well-endowed boyfriend. In new relationships, diarists are more likely to fantasize about their current partners, who are still new and exciting to them.

· ·

The Stepmom in a Hot Long-Term Relationship

42, New York City

TUESDAY

2:00 a.m.: I awake to a hard-on jabbing the back of my thighs and Jack has his hands up my tank top. I'm very tired, but also excited because this is the second night in a row that I've been woken up this way. I'm hoping it's a trend.

2:15 a.m.: After receiving a very intense manually-administrated orgasm, I take his penis into my mouth. It's not long before he tugs on my hair and I'm on my back with my knees by my ears . . . then I am flipped over. I love being taken from behind, I have the best orgasms that way.

2:17 a.m.: I have to stuff my face into the mattress because I am making too much noise. Even though our door is closed, Jack's sons' room is right next to ours and I worry they will hear.

2:45 a.m.: We're spent and cuddling, and disagreeing over who's going to go get water for the both of us, when we hear the toilet flush. Oh, shit.

9:30 a.m.: At my corporate job, having erotic flashbacks. I am still really into Jack after seven years.

12:00 p.m.: Flipping through a feminist magazine, and I see a review for a "natural" lube. I find a link on Drugstore.com and email it to Jack with the subject line, "Buy this for us!" I used to never need it, but my body no longer reacts like it used to: I find I can be horny as hell and dry as a bone. This disturbs me. I worry Jack will think I'm not sexually aroused when I am.

11:30 p.m.: Posting photos on my Facebook page, when a guy I fooled around with in high school pops up on my chat. I am super friendly and "don't get" any of his innuendos. Not flattered, because he's obviously taking the machine-gun approach, and trying every broad he knows to find a free sex chat.

11:45 p.m.: Kids are both still up. I have a hard time having the sex life I desire with kids in the house. It's difficult to let go while on full alert to any evidence that the boys might hear or interrupt us. Though I suspect the boys know what we're up to.

1:30 a.m.: Jack's hands are up my nightgown again. I am *so* tired. I press against him, so he knows I'm not rejecting him, per se. I fall back asleep.

WEDNESDAY

6:30 a.m.: He's snoring. I lightly run my fingertips from his rib cage to his hip and he moans. I put my hand down his pants and stroke him until he's totally awake. He kisses my neck while he fingers me (no lube needed today!) and we get into the "X" position so he can penetrate me while rubbing my clitoris.

6:45 a.m.: After I come, we have side sex. We like this position because it doesn't slam the headboard against the wall. He does not orgasm, however, because he happens to look at the clock and the pressure gets to him. I will take care of him later.

8:00 a.m.: Leave for work, both kids sleeping soundly (school vacation).

11:30 a.m.: More erotic flashbacks at work. We've been on a hot streak lately, and I think it's because we're no longer trying to get pregnant after confirmation that I am infertile. I thought it was my last chance to have a child of my own, and it turns out there's no chance without major medical intervention. After a mourning period, my sex drive came back with a vengeance and I've been initiating a lot more. Sex is fun again.

8:00 p.m.: Finally home after running around with the kids. While I'm food shopping, I see someone I used to bang in my twenties at Trader Joe's. We pretend we don't see each other, because it ended horribly.

8:15 p.m.: The boys have a friend over tonight. He's going to be extremely attractive when he's out of high school. I have a quick "Stiffler's Mom" fantasy, and then very deliberately push that thought *away.*

10:30 p.m.: Jack isn't home yet, the kids are in the living room. I shut the bedroom door, open the toy drawer, pull out the remote control "bullet" and look up some orgy porn on my laptop. I get off watching writhing bodies in any and every combination and the noises of sex.

12:00 a.m.: We're in bed, Jack is tired, asks me jokingly if I'd rub his back until he falls asleep. So I do.

THURSDAY

6:30 a.m.: I wake up with Jack's leg flung over my hip. I burrow into him. He rubs my lower back and I scratch his. We sort of dry hump for a minute or two and both groan. And then we get up. Time is the ultimate cockblock.

10:30 a.m.: On the phone, a friend is complaining about her lack-luster sex life with her husband. I wonder if our sex life is good because we are *not* married. Does it really make that big of a difference, mentally? I've been shacked up with him for seven years, and if anything, it's gotten better because it's deeper—there's a lot of intensity and eye contact.

5:30 p.m.: I come home from work to find Jack already home and napping in his underwear. I shut the door and lay down next to him, running my hands all over his chest and stomach and slide my hand past the waistband of his shorts. Things start to get heated and his face is between my legs when there's a pounding on the door. The older son wants to know if there's clean laundry in our room. He needs to change before heading to a music lesson. Ugh! Both very frustrated.

11:00 p.m.: There will be no finishing, because I am dead to the world.

FRIDAY

6:15 a.m.: I wake up to Jack slowly kissing me from between my shoulder blades up to the base of my neck. I enjoy it, and then roll over and straddle him. I hold the headboard so it doesn't slam against the wall, and I ride him until my eyes water. He buries his face between my breasts to muffle his moans, and both of us come pretty hard. It feels like it's been a two-day tease to get to this.

6:45 a.m.: I don't know why we bother to try to fool around any other time than the morning because that seems to be the only time we can actually fuck. He laughs and says he still likes to try.

1:00 p.m.: My primarily gay best friend forever just called to tell me that he's confused: he let a woman pick him up on his birthday, and he couldn't believe how into sex with a woman he was. I said, "Maybe you are turned on by individual people, you don't care about the actual equipment." I kind of envy that. I sometimes fantasize about sex with women, but like the orgy fantasies, they will stay in my head.

10:30 p.m.: We are in bed early because we have to get up early to drive upstate for a family reunion and sports game. We wrap around each other and try to sleep.

SATURDAY

6:00 a.m.: Up and loading the car; the boys are disgruntled.

11:00 a.m.: Surrounded by family. I stay physically close to Jack to help ease his social anxiety. My loud family can be overwhelming. When no one's looking, I squeeze his ass.

4:00 p.m.: I'm sitting in a circle of cousins and aunts and we're talking men, babies, jobs. I try not to get depressed about how I will never have my own baby. I am cradling a distant cousin. "When are you going to have one?" my Aunt asks, "It's not too late. . ." Ugh.

7:00 p.m.: Baseball game. The boys have seats in a different row than us, Jack has his hand *very* high on my inner thigh, stroking my vulva through my jeans. I hide his hand with an oversized red foam #1 souvenir hand across my lap. The game starts to get really good and Jack completely forgets about me.

1:00 a.m.: Somewhere on the highway, Jack says, "Remember when we drove back from New Hampshire?" Of course I do. He had his eyes on the road, but his hand up my skirt and made me come so hard I bit my tongue. No chance of this happening with the boys in the car.

3:30 a.m.: Home, finally. Too exhausted for anything but sleep.

SUNDAY

10:30 a.m.: Sweet, slow, sleepy morning foreplay until Jack pulls out the new lube I asked him to order. It doesn't irritate at all. He also pulls out a new toy he bought while on the website – a surprise. He orders me to hold it against my clit while he takes me from behind. Incredible, I orgasm so many times I lose count.

11:30 a.m.: Stagger to embrace Mr. Coffee. I haven't consumed alcohol in many years, but I feel like I have a hangover. We should have gotten a hotel last night, but I'm glad we didn't.

7:00 p.m.: I've been napping off and on all day. I am aware that Jack curled up with me at one point, but I wake up alone. I think he and the boys went off to forage for food.

11:00 p.m.: I have thoughts of waking Jack up for some more sex, but I very discreetly take care if it myself next to him, thinking of a dark, nasty orgy.

MONDAY

6:30 a.m.: The alarm goes off, and Jack and I spoon, cuddle, and grope each other until the last possible second and I stumble to the shower while he goes to make coffee.

1:00 p.m.: At the gym on my lunch hour—I love to look at that one personal trainer with the amazing quads.

7:00 p.m.: Coffee with a friend. We both complain about aborted sexual attempts because of kids. I'm glad I'm not alone. At least mine *knock.* Hers are still really young and just attempt to barge in, and wail if the door is locked. Both of us admit that it's fun sneaking around with that fear of being caught hanging over our heads, like when we were teenagers afraid of our parents busting us.

11:00 p.m.: Jack slides into bed next to me. We lie on our sides talking about the day. Well, I'm talking. He's kissing my neck and murmuring in my ear and making me lose my train of thought.

11:30 p.m.: I'm hanging on to the headboard, my ass is up in the air, he's pulling my hair like reins, and I'm biting my lips so I don't scream. We collapse and I rest my head on his chest until we both fall asleep.

The Sensual Lesbian Sex Educator

30, Durham, North Carolina

SUNDAY

8:35 a.m.: The first thing I want to do every morning is dive into Isabella's warm skin, her endless curves. The second thing I want to do every morning is go to the bathroom. Necessity trumps delight.

8:46 a.m.: She always wants to go back to bed and cuddle after our morning bathroom routines. How can I deny her?

9:25 a.m.: I stroke, scratch, graze her skin with featherlight pressure as she talks. I nuzzle in, finding her musky smell and sniffing it deep into my body, feeling at home. My hands go to work. Her curves always lead me back to the same place.

9:36 a.m.: When I am inside her, I think of nothing else but her pleasure, noticing the texture of the flesh on my fingers, the subtle changes of temperature, the movement of her hips, the sound of her breath. Together we orchestrate wave after wave of pleasure, as she shudders again and again. I know the only thing that will end this is my own fatigue. When I am spent I rest inside her, one hand resting on her asshole, the other just inside her pussy. Suddenly she sneezes and my hand is ejected out with great force. Laughing.

9:50 a.m.: I glance in the mirror and notice my own bright eyes. Fucking her makes me feel beautiful and powerful. It wakes up the best part of me.

12:06 p.m.: We spend most of the day naked. When I walk into the room and see her eyes light up at the sight of my naked body, it makes me feel so loved, just as I am. Her love has been a salve, helping me heal years of fat girl syndrome.

1:56 p.m.: Before I met Isabella, I was in the queer kinky poly community in California. My primary lover was an amazing transgender guy, but I frequently attended sex parties where I would touch lots of people of all genders and orientations. At the end, it no longer felt like where I was supposed to be.

2:00 p.m.: When I met Isabella, I knew, before the first kiss really, that we'd spend our lives together. Our first meal was like our thousandth. I never expected to be monogamous, but after being with her, I had no interest in sex with other people. But I'm glad we were both sluts in our twenties. I've had amazing, heart-stopping sex with men, both rough and tender. I've been with transgender men and women. I've had sex with more women than I can count. I explored BDSM to the edges. I would try anything once, twice if I didn't hate it. Those adventures allow me to know that I am satisfied. And this is where I landed: a monogamous lesbian with occasional fantasies about men.

6:05 p.m.: Cooking together. I'm shedding thirty pounds so I can become a better lover, and to prepare my body for pregnancy.

9:33 p.m.: Reading about home births. I get so excited about babies and birthing. My lover less so. I know I am being naive in my excitement about parenting, but I just can't help it. If my partner was a man, I'd have poked holes in my diaphragm months ago.

MONDAY

7:38 a.m.: The first thing I do when I wake up is check our overnight sales of our small online business. We just had our first sale in China.

11:27 a.m.: I need to start wearing more clothes. Isabella is much more prone to stay in lover mode all day. We joke about how impossible this would be if we had one more person working with us.

12:32 p.m.: Guys often ask us if we, as lesbians, sit around and touch each other's boobs all day. The answer is yes, yes we do.

4:39 p.m.: My best friend and occasional lover, Jake, died one year ago. When he comes up in conversation, I still feel brittle.

6:59 p.m.: Sometimes I feel ashamed about how happy I am. The truth is, I am fantastically happy. I feel blessed. I am doing work I love, with a woman I love. Funny thing is how hard that is to admit in public.

TUESDAY

8:19 a.m.: I need more time alone. I hate it when we fight. It never lasts long, but those moments are so ugly. We are not being our best selves.

3:18 p.m.: Lunch with a local minister who works with homeless folks. Talked about how the homeless are rarely touched. Then the conversation moved to affluent, married people who live in big houses and haven't touched in 20 years. Touch is a biological need and so many of us, rich and poor, are starving.

7:55 p.m.: One of my straight guy friends recently announced, "Fingering a girl doesn't count as sex." To which I said, "Then I haven't had sex in years!" My primary sex act is hand sex. Our hands are the most sensitive, dexterous part of our body and are capable of creating an amazing range of sensations. I love using my hands to get my lover off. I feel sad for guys who are so focused on their dicks that they miss out on other hot experiences.

7:57 p.m.: I do wonder what it would be like to have a penis to go inside my lover's body. But I love the range of sex acts we enjoy. I've mastered the art of simultaneous anal and genital stimulation—using both my hands at once to touch her entire sexual system. Oral sex, of course, has its place, in our lesbian bed. But my hands are capable of way more dexterity than any penis or dildo.

10:54 p.m.: Too tired for sex. A large plate of lunch killed my sex drive all day long. Food really makes a difference. But Isabella is craving it. She hinted several times that she'd like to make love, and she's lit candles, made the bed nicely, and spritzed rosewater. This woman means business.

11:30 p.m.: I climbed in for a cuddle. We rolled around a bit, kissed, nuzzled. As I found the energy to touch her, she responded. She is the most erotically responsive person I have ever been with. Her body moves *into* touch.

11:33 p.m.: I dove in, pressing firmly into her mons with a soft open hand. I touched her clit through her labia, slowly building to direct touch. I licked, I sucked, I bit, I kissed her all over. As I slid two fingers into her vagina and massaged her ass with the other hand, I felt her desire overflowing. How could I almost have let her go to bed with this much desire? I move my hands in rhythms that respond to her arousal, hold still after she climaxes and then slowly build up again. This is my prayer.

11:34 p.m.: After, we talked quietly and laughed.

WEDNESDAY

10:28 a.m.: Intense workout . I struggle. I look over and watch Isabella doing squats. The pleasure of watching her body in motion is much much easier to focus on.

11:23 a.m.: Chanting "Coffee, coffee!"

6:25 p.m.: Had a bit of a meltdown today. Felt so much sadness and rage about all the years of sexual abuse as a kid, and the eating disorders and shame my body experienced. I have flashes, moments where it comes back to me, and I feel like my whole life has been a reaction to the abuse. I don't feel like a victim that often. But something about working out recently has begun melting all those years down into a pool of vengeful lava. Trying to channel it into growth.

7:19 p.m.: One thing that I've never told even my best friends is how deeply I was affected by being sexually abused as a child. It's such a secret because I don't even know: it's a vicious cycle to figure out what caused what. Was I sexually promiscuous because of the abuse? Or was I abused because I was fat and therefore had breasts at age seven? I end up feeling like a strong survivor who has gained wisdom from my experiences.

8:35 p.m.: Another long day working side-by-side. We started our business three months into our relationship. Mostly it works—any issues that come up allow us to resolve issues about power dynamics or communication that would have eventually surfaced in our relationship.

8:46 p.m.: We try to exchange at least ten minutes of massage every day. Whenever I feel annoyed or tired.

8:56 p.m.: I am a much better giver than receiver. In life, and in sex. It is way harder for me to receive touch and allow myself to be taken. I am well aware of the why—sexual abuse, and personal proclivity. It takes a lot for me to feel pleasure. For years I tried to fix the numbness with heavy sensation, BDSM, high-risk situations. None of it worked very well. Now, I am trying to slow thaw.

THURSDAY

8:00 a.m.: Dreamed last night about my dead lover. I still dream about Jake all the time. Sometimes we are driving wildly in the desert, other times we are fucking like we did ten years ago. The sex I had with him was unlike anything I have experienced: it was a mix of raw and bestial, with a huge dose of friendship. My body remembers. But when I wake, I find Isabella's smooth body, and I am grateful for the veil between the living and the dead.

8:59 a.m.: Jake was also the one man I was ever in love with. We were planning on having kids together, with him as a donor. Something shifted between us, and the raw sexual energy was transformed into something sweeter. We began drinking tea together instead of vodka tonics. When he died suddenly and stupidly, my world caved in. Isabella chose to stay with me as I mourned another lover. I felt like a widow with a wife.

3:57 p.m.: Being a woman in love with a femme makes me understand a lot about straight men. Isabella just walked up and rubbed her breasts—which are the most perfect, large, full, heavy, gorgeous breasts I have ever seen—on my head. I get why men are obsessed with breasts.

They are the most perfect expressions of sensuality, one of the great masterpieces of nature.

3:58 p.m.: I grab her arm and sink my teeth into it. I like her reaction—a mixture of surprise and pain.

7:01 p.m.: Thinking about anal play. It's not a huge part of my own eroticism, but the anus is a highly erogenous zone, an integral part of the sexual system. The way porn portrays anal sex is a travesty. Hopefully people know that it can be treated with the same love and respect we (hopefully) offer to the rest of our lover's body.

10:51 p.m.: Strange to have constant low-grade anxiety about not "being enough" for the woman I love, despite the fact that she has never indicated this. When will I feel worthy of love?

FRIDAY

9:24 a.m.: I wonder how people survive offices, acting serious and professional all day long. Don't they need hugs? After working for a while, I need touch. I don't need sex or an orgasm—I need skin-to-skin contact. I pull Isabella into bed for five minutes.

3:46 p.m.: Made a big work decision. It was a tough one, but we feel complete solidarity.

7:00 p.m.: Getting ready for a picnic, watching Isabella get ready. She catches me staring.

1:59 a.m.: Bar. Bar hopping is so different at 30 years old than 25. Sober, sleepy.

2:12 a.m.: I am talking to our married friends about life with kids, and out of the corner of my eye, watch a young man and woman walk off into the night, the sexual energy palpable. I imagine they are off for a wild night of rough sex and intoxicated abandon. I crave the adventure of being single and stalking my sexual prey. I miss the feeling of fucking new people, tasting new lips. In moments like this, I need to dig deep to feel the sureness of my relationship.

SATURDAY

2:18 p.m.: I used to be able to stay up till 3 without worrying about it. Now I need to factor in an entire day of recovery. We're back in bed for a nap.

3:00 p.m.: She seduced me, scratching and biting, and bringing me to a beautiful orgasm with her mouth and fingers, allowing me to just relax and enjoy the sensations. Oral sex is a beautiful way to learn how to receive. I recently read a writer who said she found receiving oral lonely, because her lover was "all the way down there." I couldn't disagree more. It's such an intimate gift.

6:00 p.m.: We walk. Every day we walk for an hour. Something about the summer thunderstorms here in the South intoxicates me.

11:45 p.m.: I feel so blessed to do life as a team. Sometimes I am nostalgic for the anticipation of a new lover, but I am finding the sweetness of partnership to be way more daring, way more adventurous than the years of sexcapades. I look forward to that journey. ***

Partners: We're Long on Commitment and Short on Sex

After your pulse has recovered from the Lovers, you'll note what the Partners are often not getting: sex.

Partners enjoy a fantastic dynamic, filled with joy and communication and shared lives. They are held together by family, religious binds, or long-term commitment. And they are blunt about it. The Female Minister writes, "Our marriage is rooted in a strong spiritual foundation. Our relationship with each other is actually secondary to our relationship with God." In the next chapter, The Devout Grandmother writes, "I don't think of Will as my soul mate." These lines would never appear in a Lover diary.

These diarists build their intimacy through meals and trips and daily activities, and put great value on taking care of one another, particularly in life's little details: buying groceries, driving one another into town. Both diarists in this section feel fulfilled by serving their partner meals, and making sure he is well looked after—they consider it something of a duty.

And yes. Partners are the most likely to bemoan the fact that they're not having sex. Sex is only a major issue in its lack—more sexually active diarists think about it much less. You'll see a theme in Partners throughout the book: guilt, or a sense that they're falling short of sexual expectations. Which is unfortunate. Because their relationships are often happy and healthy. These diarists have made an active decision to prioritize family or religion or companionship over sex, and that's absolutely fine. Nearly half of the diaries I've read over the years fall into this category.

When Partners lament their sex lives, I want to chime in and say, "Actually, among Partners, you're absolutely normal. And you're the benefactor of a very stable life, with a spouse who enjoys living with you and shares your values." Each relationship needs to be judged on its own terms. And for these diarists, their terms are a great household and circle of friends, with consistent—though not frequent—sex. And the fact is, most do get laid *regularly*, a couple of times a month, often prescheduled. Long-term cohabitation is, in fact, the number one way to ensure consistent sex, due to easy access. Numerous sex surveys show that a mere 2 percent of marrieds are celibate.

The Female Minister writes that she's "longing to have a deeply spiritual experience from intimacy." She is one of the many Partners who poignantly senses that there's a deeper sexual and emotional relationship world than what she's experiencing. But in her decade of meeting, courting, and marrying her husband, she has never prioritized sex. What she has is a partner in life. Priorities breed realities, many of them enviable.

The Female Minister Spicing Up
Her Sex Life

30, Baltimore, Maryland

SATURDAY

8:48 a.m.: Last night my husband and I shared in our most favorite pleasure: food. I wish that instead of food we were sharing sex, but the truth is the homemade peanut brittle sounded better. I do enjoy our sex, but food has been my lover and my God far longer.

10:54 a.m.: Been thinking a lot about our intimacy issues lately. I worry constantly about my lack of desire towards physical intimacy and what that might do to our marriage. We're happily together for a decade and married for three years, attracted to each other, and enjoy a deep spiritual connection, yet I can't seem to shake this deep belief that sex is to be enjoyed by men, not women. I am longing to experience a deeply spiritual experience from intimacy.

1:46 p.m.: On my way to lunch, an 18-wheeler was driving beside me. I sped up, he sped up. I slowed, he slowed. Then I realized my skirt was hiked up really high. And so did he. Just when I was starting to think men aren't just sex-crazed pigs.

9:36 p.m.: I just performed a wedding for two people in their late twenties who revealed that tonight will be their first time. Made me wonder how it would have been different if my husband was my first.

10:00 p.m.: Can't wait to see my husband. Being as WonderBread-white as I am, I never imagined myself with anyone but a white guy. It was definitely a surprise that the man I ended up marrying was an immigrant. I would not trade my relationship with my husband for anything in this world.

11:00 p.m.: I was wondering about the "first time" thing enough to come home, have some vodka, and play pretend with the husband. The result: mind-blowing sex. Wow. I needed that.

SUNDAY

9:01 a.m.: Still glowing from last night's romp. If our intimacy could be like that all the time, we'd be set. Now if I could just get that loose without the vodka and loud music. Off to another wedding.

9:15 a.m.: I am a nonreligious minister—ordained, but it's spirituality, not dogma, that resonates.

11:30 a.m.: I hate to say it's not as special for nonvirgins, but the day isn't as layered with meaning. Today's couple is focused on the day, the flowers, the details. Yesterday those two were thinking about one thing: getting laid.

12:45 p.m.: Lunchtime. Glorious lunchtime. Which today consists of handfuls of trail mix. I think I get more pleasure out of food than sex. I look forward to it, I plan it, and it never disappoints. I often view sex as something to get through. I have never once felt like I had to get through my trail mix.

7:50 p.m.: At the gym taking "Body Pump." It's usually taught by some ridiculously skinny chic, but not today! The instructor just took off his shirt to reveal the most amazingly sexy muscles. Note to self: convince husband to take steroids.

9:00 p.m.: Evening prayer. There are three people in my marriage. My husband, myself, and God. Our marriage is rooted in a strong spiritual foundation. Our relationship with each other is actually secondary to our relationship with God. Instead of committing to "when death do us part" at our wedding we said, "as long as we both are serving our souls' highest purpose."

MONDAY

6:04 a.m.: Just awoke from a totally hot sex dream. This never happens. The details were hazy but I can say this: it was a religious experience. The message seemed to be that enlightenment through sex is possible and fun. Wondering if I should roll over and wake up the husband to find out.

5:05 p.m.: Disturbing phone call with my mother today. She told me that she needed my spiritual counsel, and then she proceeded to drop the "I think I'm going to leave your father" bomb. Can't say I blame her; he has become completely unbearable. I made the mistake of asking when they last had sex. Six months ago. She told me not to worry, she "has a toy" that she uses. File this under TMI.

9:05 p.m.: It's fair to say the conversation is consuming me. It made me remember the time my mom took me on a walk as a teen and told me that women don't like sex. She said, "Gwen, sex is something that you get through and use as a tool of manipulation. Men need it, women endure it to get what they want. Then they take care of pleasuring themselves." No wonder I am having such a hard time reinventing sex.

9:54 p.m.: Hubby is getting ready for bed. There is really nothing that I have not been honest with him about my previous sex life. He used to get really hurt by how many experiences I had that weren't with him. My husband was a virgin when we got together. He originally wasn't sure he could marry me knowing he would then never get the chance. Truth be told, I am still terrified that one day those old feelings may come back for him and he will act on them. Please, God, don't let that happen.

TUESDAY

9:01 a.m.: Just got done exercising with my hubby. I always feel so ridiculously horny after a good workout. I would never tell him that, though, because then he'd call me on it. Is it weird that I like being horny more than I like satisfying the urge? I need the horny to build up. He's ready to go anytime.

12:30 p.m.: Husband just confessed to me that he bought porn on TV a few weeks ago when I was out. *I am furious.* This makes me so mad because we've talked about this so many times. This totally pushes all of my buttons, namely that it makes me put him in the "big fat pig" category. And the fact that he waited to tell me. Need to go breathe.

4:00 p.m.: Just got an email from a client who is getting over her partner's emotional affair. She has healed a lot but just can't seem to get intimate with him again. I am giving her the textbook advice—feel her feelings, allow herself the space to heal spiritually. But honestly, if that was me, I would withhold sex forever, not just because I was wounded but because secretly I would want him to "pay for it." I have felt like this *a lot.*

7:31 p.m.: Very beautiful woman at Starbucks. Women are so physically appealing. One time in college I had the opportunity to be with a woman, but I chickened out. However, often when I fantasize while masturbating, it is about women with other women, with a man there, too. I just find it strange since when actually given the chance, it wasn't appealing.

7:38 p.m.: I do wish I had explored masturbation with vibrators and toys before I was married. I was always afraid of them, and my mom never mentioned them. I just got my first two toys eight months ago, one dildo and one little clitoris stimulator, and the little one has started to take a lead role in our sexual encounters. The big guy is still in the box. My husband is intimidated by it, and now I have his ego to worry about.

WEDNESDAY

7:50 a.m.: Cuddling with husband. He has taught me how to feel—before him I lived only in my head, and had never once enjoyed sex. He is the only guy who ever made me orgasm from oral sex, and the time he spends down there should win him an award.

10:15 a.m.: I follow the "if it isn't on my calendar, it's not happening" system. Sadly, this includes sex. Sunday is for sex. We both know this. We have both become accustomed to this and *I hate it.* I tried once to just be spontaneous . . . and we went for three weeks with no sex.

10:25 a.m.: I am annoyed at the lack of spontaneity in our sex life. Tonight I am going to surprise him. Let's just see if he can be flexible, too.

12:00 p.m.: Wow. Facebook is causing many relationship problems for couples I counsel. This year I have had five cases of infidelity by people who have reunited secretly with ex-lovers and gotten caught. Thank God I would never be tempted by my exes. They are exes because we are done. That is not the case for most.

7:00 p.m.: I am spread out on the bed in lingerie awaiting his arrival. A new goal: in a year from now, I hope to have the official "my wife is freaking hot and a sex kitten" title. When not ministering, that is.

8:09 p.m.: Success. He was definitely quite pleasantly surprised to say the least. The verdict: I am definitely the one with the spontaneity issue. He was totally ready to go. He asked zero questions. And it was gooood. ***

Religious diarists frequently land in stable, low-but-consistent sex Partnerships. This tracks with national statistics: regular churchgoers have 25 percent less sex than the national average, and a full quarter of churchgoers are celibate, nearly double the national average.[2] Yet many of these marriages are quite successful, populated by diarists who naturally blossom through the ritual and structure of marriage, religion, and husband/wife roles.

The Obedient Fundamentalist Military Wife is among the most revelatory diaries in the book. Her marriage is on the conservative side of the 20 percent of evangelical U.S. marriages, the inner workings of which are usually secreted, out of fear that honesty about sex is not in the service of the marriage. (She repeatedly stressed to me that she did not want to embarrass her husband.) Her husband and marriage are the two pillars of her world, and so her focus is on how to serve both, and she gets great satisfaction out of being useful and appreciated. Self-discovery as an individual isn't particularly relevant to that world view, and is in fact potentially damaging to her marriage; instead, she conceives of herself as part of a union.

In the course of her diary, she takes marital advice about scenarios that have yet to arise, from both a radio program and a stranger at the church. She can do this because her marriage has an outside structure to it, giving her a sense of how she "should" behave long before actual situations happen. When she responds to her husband, her responses are almost predetermined. (The Female Minister does the same thing, launching into a predecided response when she discovers that her husband has again ordered porn.) "There is truly freedom within the boundaries of marriage," she writes. Her "freedom" lies in the fact that while other diarists spend pages (and pages) writing some version of "Oh, no, what should I do?" she is free of that. She has a path; her issue is just staying on it . . . and praying that her husband does too.

If the Lover diaries are about flexibility, immediacy, and intimacy, the Partner diaries are about structure. Each couple intrinsically agrees upon a predetermined path, and fills their days with little gestures affirming the path: greetings, farewells, errands for one another, coffee, kisses on the cheek, and yes, once-a-week sex.

The Obedient Fundamentalist Military Wife Who Would Like More Sex, Please

30, Anchorage, Alaska

THURSDAY

8:38 a.m.: Women in Alaska have a saying about men: "The odds are good, but the goods are odd." This is a man's paradise, with all of the fishing, hunting, boating, snow-machining, and four-wheeling. I'm glad Alaska is only our temporary home while my husband is in the military. But I'm also glad he's having his fun.

8:41 a.m.: My husband just left for work. I am so sore—I had oral surgery a couple of days ago. I can't believe I'm stumbling around the kitchen, making coffee. I'm happy I can do this for him—it's our morning routine—but I can't wait to sit.

8:53 a.m.: My husband cc's me in an email. One of his relatives is stumbling out of the faith, getting addicted to drugs and alcohol, without a job, divorced with two kids, and continually making mistakes, like DUI. We pray for them every day. I'm so grateful my husband makes good decisions and is faithful to a Christian God.

9:00 a.m.: Just thinking that my husband was so sweet before he left, calling me beautiful even though I'm all swollen, gently kissing me, and making sure I was set for the day. He randomly told me he loved me before we fell asleep last night—I love those surprise "I love yous." We've been married over a year, and I am a lucky girl. I do worry that things won't always be this way, though.

9:05 a.m.: Shower and think about my husband's booty, which I snuck a peak of as he was getting ready for work. Well, not so snuck. When he came out of the shower, I'm pretty sure I grabbed it and gave it a smack. Ha, ha! I once left a note in his underwear drawer: "I love your cute, tight butt!"

12:11 p.m.: My husband calls to check in. He offers to come home early to make me something easy to eat. I am high on Percocet. Groggy.

8:00 p.m.: My husband came home from work, and took me out to eat with friends. He made sure I had food I could eat, put his arm around me during dinner, and drove back and forth so I wouldn't have to worry about it.

10:00 p.m.: We snuggled up on the couch to watch TV; he helped me upstairs when I was falling asleep. I love him so much.

10:30 p.m.: A secret: My husband and I don't have sex very often. A normal week is once, maybe twice. Since we are newlyweds, I'd just expected more. This is a big secret. Actually, I did tell my very best friend, and now am at peace. She suggested it was a personality thing. Her husband has a job filled with others' problems, and they have sex every night! She thinks it's because he likes that comfort. My husband likes a strict schedule. Often we plan a day or two ahead of time to have sex; I think it mentally prepares him. He likes to eat and relax with TV. Sometimes this angers me—shouldn't he prioritize his wife over TV? But when I've expressed my concerns, he's always quick to make me a priority. We are still learning how to make sex a more prominent part of our schedule, if we want that. Like most things, I've learned to not sweat it, and to take opportunities as they arise.

FRIDAY

7:52 a.m.: My husband tells me about a nightmare he had: We were on a boat, and somehow I fell into the water and a shark grabbed me. He had a pistol and he jumped in after me. He shot the shark in the head, twice, but every time he shot him it just grabbed me tighter. My husband has nightmares where he is unable to protect me. I'm flattered that this is a nightmare for him. Sometimes I am resentful of the things he asks me not to do, like running when the streets are icy, but I am grateful when I realize that it's for my protection and he doesn't want to see me hurt.

7:54 a.m.: I say, "But you woke up, and I'm right here, Babe!" He jokingly tells me that when I pull back the covers, my legs are gonna be gone. Ack! Haha—we're so funny.

10:49 a.m.: We had our shower routine again this morning: he steps out naked, I grab his butt. He hisses like a cat. I laugh and grab his butt again. Then he gives me a gentle slap on my rear. It's these comfortable-with-each-other married scenes that I was longing for before I got married. I never knew how good they'd feel.

11:38 a.m.: I'm on the couch again today, so I'll tell you a bit about me: I was raised Roman Catholic, but as I grew, I identified increasingly more as a Protestant Christian. Mostly I switched because I wanted to live like the faithful Christians in the Protestant church I attended. Eventually, through friends there, I met my husband.

11:48 a.m.: For many Christians, marriage is a no-brainer—Christians marry Christians, or else part of one's faith is compromised. I dated a Jewish guy in high school, and our relationship would never work, because I needed to date a Christian guy who would be motivated by his faith to avoid the temptations that others embrace, like porn, infidelity, or fornication. I couldn't change his mind; only his loyalty to God could keep him faithful. My husband's fundamental values are the same as mine, and that's what makes our marriage work.

11:55 a.m.: Before my husband, I had one consistent hook up in college. In the big city when I lived alone, I was scared to date men, for fear I would be obligated to have sex. I'd been skating along, hoping to meet the right person. For about ten years before I was married, I struggled with not being married, and wondering if I ever would. I continued praying to God to give me a husband. After two years of searching, we were introduced long distance, and after the first weekend, we decided to get married. Contemporary society says that people need to live together and have sex before committing their lives to each other. I'll be blunt: that is crap. That method is selfish and offensive to God. I didn't need to be in a relationship before I learned how to be in this one; I know how to be in one now because I love my husband. God puts us in the right place at the right time for a reason, and this reason was to marry my husband.

11:58 a.m.: The only person I have had sex with is my husband. I am thrilled about that, for both our sakes. He never had to worry about someone in my past. I never had to worry about pregnancy or STDs. We have learned to be comfortable with each other, and are learning to please each other. There is truly freedom within the boundaries of marriage.

1:48 p.m.: Percocet again, woozy. My husband texts to tell me he is bored, and he wishes he was with me.

4:35 p.m.: I text Husband to say our friend is picking me up. He likes me to check in. Before we met, I didn't care about answering my cell. But my husband expected me to always be able to hear it, answer it, or text back. I had to learn to respect his wishes; he's learned there are times when I can't (in the shower, in an interview) and to be patient. I promised him I would always make his calls a priority.

5:30 p.m.: We go out to a steakhouse. I can't help looking around for my husband so I can make a decision about what to eat. He wouldn't want me to eat something chewy because my mouth is still healing. I keep my phone out.

6:03 p.m.: Husband calls; he's on his way. He asks for a Crown & Coke and a glass of water. The waitress doesn't show up for 10 minutes, and I get anxious. I really want it on the table when he gets there. I like to please him.

6:30 p.m.: Husband shows up, drinks are on the table. I feel pleased with myself for making that happen.

6:31 p.m.: Lobster bisque is delicious; the best thing I've had all week. Husband admonishes me for chewing on a piece of bread. Whoops, I guess I shouldn't have eaten that, considering my situation.

8:30 p.m.: Home. I'm out of my head from the Percocet, margatini, and vodka soda. Cuddle for husband's nightly TV wind-down.

9:40 p.m.: Feel dizzy, like I'm about to pass out. I tell Husband. He immediately shuts off the TV, gathers up our things, and helps me upstairs.

SATURDAY

9:00 a.m.: My daily take-your-birth-control cell alarm goes off. We're training for a half marathon, and Saturdays are our long run days. Last night Husband suggested we run early. I am doubtful; he's snuggled in pretty peacefully next to me. I call it "morning squeeze." Cute.

10:20 a.m.: Wandering around the house, lazily preparing for this run.

11:00 a.m.: Finally, driving to a scenic trail I like to run. I'm nervous because last time we ran nine miles I struggled, and because I had to convince Husband of this trail—if he doesn't like it, I'll be hearing about it. I tell Husband I am nervous and he encourages me. He puts his hand on my thigh while we drive. I feel better, but I won't feel totally better unless the run goes well.

11:15 a.m.: Running. I can feel my jaw, but it doesn't hurt. Now I just have to run nine miles.

11:30 a.m.: I announce that I want to run up the huge hill at the end. He discourages this idea, says it's not necessary, but I think he might be lazy. I tell him I'm going to do it; he doesn't stop me. It's a strategy I've learned with him: tell him beforehand so he can make plans about it, then he's usually agreeable. I'm glad I spoke my mind.

12:40 p.m.: In the last three miles, Husband hurts my feelings. My knee is hurting, and he tells me we shouldn't run up that hill at the end. Ugh, why does he tell me this now? I thought we already agreed! I argue with him, tell him I still intend to do it. He says, "You can't even keep up the pace that we had in the beginning," then he speeds up and leaves me. This often happens—he gets stressed and says something mean, and I spend the last two miles running alone.

1:00 p.m.: He makes up for hurting my feelings by meeting me at the hill and running it with me. I tell him he hurt my feelings. He doesn't immediately apologize, but he defends himself. That is so annoying. Just say you are sorry! We make up.

1:25 p.m.: I need to eat something. He wants to run errands. As we wait to get the car washed, I have to put my head between my legs because I feel so sick. Finally, he feels bad about me feeling bad. We're almost home, he says.

1:40 p.m.: We get home, I eat, and he is in a good mood. All is well in our household.

6:00 p.m.: Husband watched basketball all afternoon, and fixes me some yummy pasta for dinner.

8:00 p.m.: I find I like to be alone for 2–3 hours, and then I need to hear from him. If I'm gone from him for too long, he'll come looking for me. I come downstairs.

10:03 p.m.: I'm sitting in bed working on the computer (I work from home), and Husband is reading. Suddenly he stops, puts the book down, and then turns to snuggle with me. This is our joke because he always does it unexpectedly. I smile inside when he grabs me. We snuggle for a while, tell each other I love you, and fall asleep.

3:00 a.m.: My mouth hurts so much. I'm awake taking medicine. It didn't hurt during our long run. I'm worried.

SUNDAY

7:30 a.m.: He's got morning wood. I enjoy teasing him about that, but this morning my sore jaw makes me forget.

8:30 a.m.: Our friends call! Husband's friends; this is the first time I am speaking to them, but I am relieved to know that they are nice. In a few months we are moving to a new base, and then my husband will be deployed, so it's nice to make connections.

9:00 a.m.: We found out about his deployment abruptly, unexpectedly, and recently. When I first heard, I got teary-eyed. But in the next few days, I got excited. It will be an opportunity to go to the big city and visit my old friends. But then I felt so guilty about wanting to go back to my old life. I think this deployment will be an opportunity for me to explore the new location where we'll be stationed. I have to remember that my old life is part of my past, not something I want to return to.

11:19 a.m.: In writing this, I've been thinking about a wife's need to please her husband. I think that's a woman's job—to observe her husband, know what he likes, and give him what he likes. Biblically, Eve was created to be Adam's helper. I think contemporary women may shun this, maybe selfishly. Well, husbands are commanded to love their wives, too. I'm not in some stodgy role, saying "yes sir" to everything. No, I am adventurous and colorful and we have balance. I tell him when I am offended, and we work it out. Pleasing people has always been part of my nature. There is harmony in the household when husbands and wives assume biblical roles, in contrast to many contemporary households, where a woman may take control, and the man is left impotent, without power, and useless.

11:38 a.m.: I look forward to the Lord's Day because I know I'll get extra hugs. I think it's because he doesn't have to stress about work today, and because he is thankful to God to have me in his life.

1:00 p.m.: Husband home from church. We listen to a sermon while he makes pancakes.

2:15 p.m.: The sermon was about raising children wisely. We discuss: how will we keep our future children out of trouble without sheltering them? He was once rebellious. We end our discussion staring out blankly from the couch.

5:15 p.m.: At a friend's booth at a fair. A couple married for 19 years comes up. They are wasted, and this makes them incredibly fun. I wonder if my husband and I will be like this couple 19 years from now. I hope so.

9:07 p.m.: Home, bedroom. Husband reasons that we can't have sex because the antibiotics lessen the effectiveness of my birth control, and he doesn't want to risk my having our first child while he's deployed. He's more excited about kids than me. He'd be devastated not to be there!

10:00 p.m.: Husband sleeping. He keeps hinting that he wants a blow job, and sometimes I start to give him one, but I've never finished one (we finish with sex). I'm nervous about how the semen will taste. What if it's gross? Yuck! I am curious to try new things, but I think I need a book or something. I don't have the imagination to dream things up! I think that we just need more time together in bed. I am working on encouraging this.

11:53 p.m.: A note about birth control: a lot of Christians shun it, a lot use it. Preachers have told us that the Bible doesn't say no to birth control, so that means it is up to prayer and thoughtfulness. The Bible does talk a lot about children as blessings. So having children is extremely encouraged. Husband's view is that we need to have them responsibly. Initially, I didn't want to be on birth control. But I am to obey my husband in his federal* decisions. So far, I'm thankful we didn't have a child immediately, because it took us a couple of months to adjust to living together.

MONDAY

6:30 a.m.: Back to normal work routine. Husband hops out of bed and gets naked. Ha ha, I love that. I love that we can just walk around naked, without shame.

8:00 a.m.: Christians speak about wives being submissive to their husbands. Faithful submission does not mean that Christian wives get bossed around. Instead, wives are submissive to their husband's federal headship. That means that a wife might give her opinion, but she submits to her husband's decision. Conversely, husbands are commanded to love their wives, which means being gentle and polite with them, always caring for them, and sacrificing for them. Because husbands are commanded to love, everything balances out. Marriage works really well by this design, God's design.

11:36 a.m.: I like that we share our car. In the car he's a captive audience and I sometimes save my thoughts for the car. Shower time is a good time to speak to him, too.

11:40 a.m.: Husband and I got some really good advice from a book about marriage that we studied together before we wed. The pastor who wrote it said that arguments and offenses are like dropping something on the carpet. The more arguments that go unresolved and offenses that go unapologized for, the more things drop on the carpet.

---

* Federal headship: In fundamentalist Christianity, the husband leads his wife and family with full authority, under a covenant with a higher power.

And so the marriage is left with a big mess. If you resolve every argument, there's never a mess. I try to live by it. In the end I'm serving God by keeping a peaceful marriage.

12:00 p.m.: Doctor's office, nervous. I have to get my annual pap smear, and my doctor is male. This is military health care. It's free, but our choices are limited. I feel uncomfortable.

12:20 p.m.: Doctor walks in with a male student-doctor. Oh, boy, the student is doing the breast exam and the pap. AGH!

12:22 p.m.: I just try to relax. There is a young nurse in the room, and I look at her for solidarity, but she looks terrified. It's more awkward, longer, and uncomfortable than I remember. I know if my husband were here he would be pissed. He can't stand the thought of other men touching me.

4:00 p.m.: After a financial adviser appointment, I race over to the base to get Husband. He tells me about his day, and I try to be encouraging. This is an important wife role, cheerleader.

7:03 p.m.: I've got a deadline looming, but Husband wants to watch a season finale. I want to see it, and Husband doesn't like it when my work gets in the way. I've made a commitment to schedule my daytime around my husband. It's part of my duty as a wife to support him, and I can't do that if I'm off doing my own thing. So I just tell myself I'll be up late.

12:22 a.m.: Still working. The finale was a letdown. I wish I was in bed with my husband! Why did I leave this until now?

2:24 a.m.: Gratefully crawl into bed, relieved to be done. Try not to wake Husband, but do anyway.

TUESDAY

7:30 a.m.: Every morning, my husband dramatically exits the shower by pulling the curtain fast and wide to reveal his tall, handsome, dripping wet naked body. He doesn't do this for effect; it's just his style to be forceful, but it stunned me the first time. It's so dramatic that I still take notice. I usually make some sort of dramatic applause, or try to grab his penis. More butt-smacking and boob-grabbing.

8:19 a.m.: Upon morning inspection, it looks like my husband used last evening to get things done—there is laundry in the wash, and the dishwasher was run. Nice.

9:17 a.m.: I run errands, getting ready for tomorrow's camping trip. I am a machine! I feel so accomplished.

12:45 p.m.: I go to transfer funds. The bank accounts aren't linked, and it will take a week. Crap crap crap. Husband will be disappointed if the plan we agreed on fails. Come up with a new plan, but I have to get approval from Husband first. He calls back, sounds happy with my new plan, and is very pleased I met our grocery budget. Yay!

1:00 p.m.: Lunch, clean up the dining room. I like to have some housework done every day when Husband comes home. It shows him that I care about the house.

3:00 p.m.: Done cleaning. Phew. Meet Husband. We are happy to see each other, and go get gas, propane, and beer. I finish the financial paperwork, and tell Husband where to sign.

7:00 p.m.: Done eating, and it's time to close up the camper. Husband has had a few beers by this time and he's muttering curses. Eeek. He's really good about not taking it out on me, except for one little quip. Finally we get it all done, get the camper in the garage, and he's magically affectionate with me.

10:31 p.m.: Husband comes up to go to bed. I ask him—sex? I'm not expecting it, and good thing, cause he says no. He's just too drunk. That's okay. We don't have any condoms. So I give him some affection and he crashes.

1:27 a.m.: Before our marriage, Husband talked a lot about all the sex we would have—in the morning, after showering, in the evening, etc. He still mentions sex a couple times a day. But we don't actually have a whole lot of sex. I think, when we decide to have kids, sex will have more of a purpose, and we'll be excited about it. Writing about it makes me think we should make it a priority. ***

Aspirers: We Have an Understanding

What is this couple's understanding? That's the question I ask whenever encountering Aspirers, to hash out their agreement, unspoken or spoken, of the goals they'd like to achieve. "Sex is the glue," writes The Sexy-Stay-at-Home Mother. Sex is a key marriage expectation, and she works hard to keep it frequent and enjoyable; she also expects her husband to financially support the household. If either were to go awry, their marriage would be shaken to its core; conversely, she has held on through many rough patches by keeping her eye on her goals.

Which is to say that the shape of Aspirer relationships is a mirror of the couple's shared goals. I published a 2010 British book of diaries which included a memorable diary from The Grandmother Who Would Like a Good Romp in the Fields, a mother of three who prioritized childrearing above all, and thirty years later, awakes to the reality that her sex life is dead on arrival. Of course it is. It was never a goal.

Many Aspirers are goal-oriented people, a habit that spills over into all aspects of their lives. They tend to be very focused parents, and when sex is a goal of their relationship, they are amusingly good at concentrating on it—witness the efforts of The Sexy Stay-at-Home Mother of Three to find adult time. Aspirers are also very focused on the big, long-term picture: The Sexy Stay-at-Home Mom knows that small children are temporary, and that she will eventually have her sex life back. For Lovers who live in the *now*, these same conditions would be intolerable.

Another theme throughout the book: Aspirers often have a best friend with whom they are closer than their partner. Which isn't to say that their relationship with their partner is flawed; it's more that Aspirer relationships are built on achieving long-term goals, to which immediate emotional honesty isn't always productive. In fact, it can be detrimental—when The Sexy Stay-at-Home Mom arrives home to find that none of her children have been fed and her husband is playing video games, she takes a deep breath, and lets the moment pass. She knows that expressing her ire will not help the kids get to bed (and, in a decade, out of the house), and her hubby into bed with her that night; and sure enough, she enjoys her evening. The result is that the level of moment-to-moment truth she's living with is a little lower. Compare this to Lover couples, to whom in-the-moment connection and honesty are paramount; they tend to find Aspirer relationships both baffling and not "real."

You can see in the pages ahead that Aspirer relationships flourish when both partners hold up their ends of the deal; these bonds are also quite good at withstanding life's financial and logistical challenges, like house hunting and child crises.

The Sexy Stay-at-Home Mother of Three

35, Faulkner County, Arkansas

WEDNESDAY

6:00 a.m.: My husband kisses me and leaves for work. Still don't get why he leaves so early. He doesn't have to be there until seven.

7:57 a.m.: Got the kids off to school. I tried to lay back down, but the four year-old, Zakera, gave me her, "[*Sigh.*] *Mommy, I love you.*" How can I not go make her breakfast after that?

1:32 p.m.: Texting my husband. I tell him that P90X, a new workout I've been doing, has my entire body sore, except for one spot. Can he come home early so we can work on it?

1:33 p.m.: Husband's leaving early.

3:39 p.m.: Husband and I just wasted two hours hanging out. What a waste of an empty house.

4:34 p.m.: Instead of taking the kids home from school, I'm dropping them at my sister's. Husband and I need a do-over.

6:00 p.m.: Talking with husband about how we never seize the moment. And guess what? He accused me of not initiating sex. WTF? I texted saying I wanted sex. What do I need to do, stand in the garage naked?

7:00 p.m.: Further discussion. Conclusion: neither of us is good at initiating sex. So we yelled and made up and then talked and then fucked. He is so good in bed. It's nice to be so vocal during sex, and not worry about the kids hearing.

7:30 p.m.: He is in the living room playing Call of Duty, and I'm Facebooking. How romantic.

7:38 p.m.: Kids are home. Duty calls. My teenager needs to talk, my grade schooler feels like she is forgotten, and my preschooler just stepped in dog shit.

11:31 p.m.: I love my children, but I can't wait for them to be old enough to send somewhere so I can do Daddy in peace.

1:16 a.m.: Just got off Chatroulette.com, a website that men go to jack off on, apparently. I went only because my friend told me about it. Kinda gross.

1:17 a.m.: I wonder if my hubby will smell my pheromone perfume, and get a hard-on and wake up and do me, like he did three times last week?

THURSDAY

10:15 a.m.: Lying here wondering how much longer my daughter will be asleep, and my husband at the dentist. Thinking of trying a new toy I ordered. Last night I couldn't bear to wake him up.

10:20 a.m.: I walk in the living room and guess who is there playing Call of Duty? He's cooked himself breakfast. And not considered the other people in the house. Men! What the hell?

11:29 a.m.: I think I live my live vicariously through soap operas. I guess that's why I expect my husband to come in and throw me down and rip off my clothes. I could text him instructions and he still wouldn't.

1:10 p.m.: Doorbell rings. It is FedEx. I needed that package—customers have been calling. I sell sex toys part time. I allow my regular customers to come by to shop whenever they need anything. Sometimes I feel like a drug dealer, meeting people in the Kroger parking lot. It's funny.

2:28 p.m.: I am so excited about the new product. One customer just left, and another is heading over.

3:00 p.m.: Oh, my God, it is so hot outside. Me and heat do not mix. It makes me mean. I cussed three people in traffic.

6:30 p.m.: Just got back from running all over town, meeting four new customers.

7:30 p.m.: Sitting outside my daughter's dance class. Yesterday when we had sex, I spotted. I should tell him I'm not really on my period, otherwise I may not get any for seven days.

7:45 p.m.: Just realizing that my sexual forecast for the weekend sucks. He's switching back to nights. Ugh. I hate his work schedule. I call his job "Kimberly," his girlfriend. I hate Kimberly.

1:38 a.m.: Just took a bath with my preschooler who never sleeps. Doesn't bother me because she'll sleep all day tomorrow and I can get some things done.

2:00 a.m.: I would love for him to roll over and fondle me. I know that won't happen. He probably fears he will end up red-handed. I remember when we use to have a lot of sex. We still do compared to most couples. We both have agreed that sex is the glue that keeps us together. It works for us. We decided once that the next time we had a disagreement we would both come in the bedroom and get butt naked. Sure enough, neither of us stays mad any more.

2:01 a.m.: We have been together a dozen years, yet only married recently. We argued some kinda terrible the year before we got married—mostly because we are both so needy, and can be real assholes. I was ready to give up on the relationship. But hands down our sex can't compare to any of our past lovers. So to us that is LOVE.

2:38 a.m.: Just to clarify: Our kids will one day grow up and be out of our house, and then we will still be having amazing sex with each other, and that glue will keep us together. Which is more than what I can say for some. Our sex is, and always has been, amazing.

FRIDAY

1:15 p.m.: Lying naked in bed and talked with my husband most of the morning. I woke him with some amazing face (our term for oral sex). He was shocked and happy. Listening to his moans and grunts only made me get more into it. He's been smiling ever since.

2:00 p.m.: We're in the same room with Zakera, the preschooler. With our laptops, we are talking dirty about how we are gonna get naked later. We are a great Facebook couple. We flirt on each others' posts.

7:00 p.m.: Went to happy hour with my cousin. Yes, I took my preschooler to happy hour. TGIFriday's. It was fun. If I don't enjoy adult time every once in a while, I feel like I'm losing my mind.

11:29 p.m.: Oldest daughter made it home safe from a party. I have talked to her about sex and STDs. We have talked about fingering, anal sex; and penises, erect, circumcised, and noncircumcised. One night we got on the Internet and looked at a website with nothing but penises on it, of all shades, sizes, colors, even ones with STDs. I think I grossed her out, and killed her curiosity. Which was exactly what I wanted to do.

11:32 p.m.: She goes to church school. A few years ago I told her that God put us here to procreate, through the covenant of marriage. She was about 11. She quickly said, "So you sinned because you and Daddy had sex before marriage." Then she started naming off people in the family that had. I told her yes, but you don't get to judge them. Only God can. That is between them and God.

12:00 a.m.: My husband's working tonight. I really hate sleeping alone. I guess I will let the preschooler sleep with me. At least it will keep me from getting bored and masturbating.

SATURDAY

2:47 p.m.: Sleeping on couch, after getting up at 6:00 a.m. for the girls' activities. Don't want to disturb my husband, who has to get up for work soon. Zakera keeps coming over, stroking my head and saying how much she loves me. Really sweet. Yet I want to scream, "Leave me the hell alone, girl!"

4:49 p.m.: So my husband leaves for work, and all these weird suspicions start entering my head. Happens every time we see each other less. Now I have to play back in my head the hundreds of reasons he would never do anything to jeopardize our relationship. But I can't help but wonder. I find myself punishing him for what someone else put me through in a previous relationship.

7:11 p.m.: The last time I was sexually aroused was 36 hours ago. That was when I awoke my husband by sucking his dick. That's so easy to type, but sounds so vulgar.

7:12 p.m.: A guy I used to date would whisper, "Suck my dick" in my ear. Oh, my God, what a turnoff. I was like, "WHAT THE HELL? Who says that? No!"

8:15 p.m.: Facebook friend's every post is about "letting God in," or "letting go" or a Bible quote. Somewhere in there, you need to fart or fry a chicken wing or drop the F-bomb in traffic. Just sayin'. Unfriended.

3:00 a.m.: Texting my husband that I am imagining him rubbing my butt like he always does. He says, "Funny, I was thinking about rubbing your butt." I love that dude!

SUNDAY

9:45 a.m.: Realize I haven't showered in two days. Jump out of bed thinking I don't want my husband to roll over and try to snuggle with me, and me smell like a dead body. Shower, bank, and post office I go.

11:54 a.m.: Talking to customers and placing orders. I didn't even have a party this weekend and made almost $300.

9:37 p.m.: Home after meeting some women to sell products to. Husband looks like he has not moved from that video game, the middle one is starving and hasn't had her bath, and the preschooler is "checking on her ABCs," which is her social networking. I have customers to answer, but no one has had dinner. I could bitch and complain, but that will only mean that I'll end up so mad that at the end of the night I won't get any.

11:24 p.m.: My husband and I are cracking up laughing, watching one of our favorite reality shows, *Tough Love Couples* on VH1. We're kissing a lot. Kids are fed and in the bed. Except the preschooler, of course. I'm so glad I didn't bitch before.

4:00 a.m.: Tried a new sex toy with my husband, which was amazing. It was a couple's toy. I wanted to scream like I was being forced into a realm of pure ecstasy. He didn't get as much out of it.

4:02 a.m.: I should do a commercial for this thing. My husband would be the man sitting next to me just nodding.

4:08 a.m.: What we just did was sex. Sex usually has oral sex and a lot of position changes, and is loud. You break a sweat. When "making love," you do more looking at each other, slow sensual movement. It usually has light moaning, as much touching as possible. "Doing it" is like a nooner. One position, just go until he comes. "Having sex" is that roll over in the middle of the night when you realize he has a hard-on, so you know it's your civic duty to handle it. Sometimes it's awkward because you really just wanna make the hard-on go down.

MONDAY

10:20 a.m.: Fell asleep naked in bed with husband, with the door locked. Awoke naked lying next to Zakera. There is something so wrong with that.

10:21 a.m.: Rolling self in the sheets like a burrito.

11:00 a.m.: Husband back from orthodontist appointment. Suggest that the next time he leaves me in bed naked and alone, lock the door.

11:30 a.m.: I hear, "Moooommmy! Jasmine is looking at the nasty stuff!" I dive into the living room, thinking I left a box out . . . and she's reading *Men's Health* magazine. I say, "No, baby, it's just a half-naked girl in a magazine."

3:15 p.m.: Planning for a toy party this weekend. I can count on one hand how many parties my husband has missed. He usually hangs out in a separate room til the party is over (unless it's couples or coed). He drives, unpacks, packs up. People always say, "He must really love you." We love the drives back. I am usually counting money, and we are cracking up at how the party went.

10:45 p.m.: Post-workout shower, enjoyed my removable shower head, and now I'm laid across the bed on a towel. I'm too tired to dry off. My husband is enjoying the view, I think.

12:34 a.m.: I should try this drying off thing more often. We kissed for what seemed like hours. Kissing is so important in a relationship. Trust me, it's not something you get if you're just sex buddies. Then sex. I think I used to be ashamed of using lubes. Now I realize it has to do with so many things. If I use my removable showerhead, like I often do, the water dries me out. We just made love, by the way.

5

recommitting

ROUND TWO

My wife said her wildest sexual fantasy would be
if I got my own apartment.

—Rodney Dangerfield

Forget about those "just the two of us" relationships, where weekend
mornings are spent staring headily into each other's eyes, and messing
with the dog or cat. The diarists in this chapter are lucky if they sleep
past 6:45 a.m., because their lives—and therefore relationships—are
heavily populated: The Retiree Who Loves His Second Wife More
Than Sex keeps tabs on seven children, a former spouse, and a small
army of grandchildren; The Gay Dad with a Hot New Boyfriend is
thoroughly occupied with an ex-wife in rehab, two kids, and a new
flame an hour away. Recommitment: it's just like commitment, with
slightly more sex, and much more baggage. Forty percent of new
American marriages are remarriages.

If one trait has jumped out at me from the hundreds of recommit-
ment diaries, it's that the relationships tend to be more extreme: The
Retiree has accepted a celibate marriage; The Self-Employed Family
Man is comfortable with very little adult time with his wife; The Gay
Dad doesn't mind seeing his boyfriend just once a week. It's because

these self-aware diarists are focusing on one or two narrow relationship priorities. Each diarist knows from experience exactly which priorities they need fulfilled in a relationship, which are superfluous, and which are best fulfilled by friends and family. These are *not* diarists who happened to meet someone great, and fell into a broadbased, loosely defined second marriage. Many have survived arduous breakups, and are conscious of their own needs, intentionally creating the relationships that they want.

An aside: Because the relationships ahead are more focused, they accentuate the pros and cons enjoyed by each relationship type—because it's utterly obvious which needs are getting met by the relationship, and which are not. An unavoidable conclusion of the diaries is that every relationship has priorities. And with priorities come non-priorities—no couple has it all, and all diarists are pushing some enviable qualities out of their lives. I often tell people that relationships are like businesses: every business has two or three services that they offer well. Not twenty-five. And the stronger and clearer those services are, the better the business will fare. The focused diarists in this chapter are down to one or two. Which is why many diaries in this book chronicle joyful, deep, fulfilling partnerships, while also documenting a host of unmet, less important needs that inevitably fall through the cracks.

	Typical Pros	Typical Cons
Lovers	• A passionate, honest, emotionally-connected partner.	• Lack of day-to-day logistical support • Ample time spent processing • Large practicality challenges
Partners	• A committed partner in life who is utterly devoted.	• Limited emotional immediacy • Fear of growing distant • Less sex
Aspirers	• An ally with whom to build a life and face the world day-to-day.	• Dishonesty or infidelity • Sense that a partner doesn't always "get" them

It's a dependably amusing sport to read the diaries with an eye toward what diarists *aren't* getting from their relationships. Diarists who understand their relationship's pros and cons are more able to fill their lives with friends and family who fulfill the missing needs, a skill that diarists in second and third unions excel at.

Partners

Fun fact: The Devout Grandma is the only handwritten diary of the book, written in cursive on stationary, and mailed. It is also an archetype of a mature second Partner relationship: She is striving for contentment, not ecstasy and she appreciates that she's alive and has a pleasant husband—the rest is water under the bridge. The aims are different than in previous relationships, where sex and compatibility and excitement were paramount.

Not surprisingly, sexual challenges are frequent among this demographic. The Retiree Who Loves His Second Wife More Than Sex is far from alone. A full third of married people over 70 are celibate, a result of old age and lack of prioritizing sex. If you think about it, it's quite odd that older diarists still pressure themselves to have consistent sexual intercourse, given that they're long past the procreative age, and the equipment no longer lends itself to the deed. Failing to maintain the same sexual appetite one had at 23 is not a dysfunction. The many diarists who decry their lack of intercourse are saying more about their conceptions of what "sex" is than about their sex lives. Male diarists are more likely to have stopped the sex, which tracks with research: in two out of three celibate marriages, it's the man who stops the sex. Both diarists ahead refer to Viagra, which while a godsend to some, has also widely spread the impression that intercourse is the only and best kind of sex—which is untrue. (See the sex life of The Sensual Lesbian Educator.)

In fact, sexual dysfunction is so stunningly common that it's not really dysfunction at all, among any age group. It's normal. Thirty-one percent of men and 43 percent of women report "at least one episode of sexual dysfunction of several months' duration" in the last year, and a third of men cop to frequent premature ejaculation. Which means that pretty much everyone experiences it in their bed.[1] The idea that intercourse equates to sex is particularly dangerous for youth, by negating "outercourse" options, which many public health experts have pointed out, would decrease STDs and teen pregnancy, and increase orgasms across the board.[2]

The Retiree is clearly suffering from his perception that sex is gone from his life forever. "I think it's particularly difficult for men, with the masculine image of the roaring, throbbing hard-on," says sexologist Dr. Betty Dodson. Dodson is vehement about the need to redefine sex, particularly in old age. "The procreative model of a penis inside of a vagina is America's fetish. There are so many things you can do that are intimate, which connect you. One of the bonuses of being a woman is that the clitoris stays viable to the very end." She adds, "If there's a biological urge to penetrate, you can use dildos." Few diarists are aware of the many options, including The Retiree.

The Retiree Who Loves His Second Wife More than Sex

81, Sarasota County, Florida

FRIDAY

7:55 a.m.: Another morning of a hug and kiss before getting out of bed. Nothing sexual about that. It has become rote.

12:02 p.m.: This morning was like every other morning: I had breakfast and read the newspaper while Nancy did her crossword puzzle. Then I left to play golf. When I got home Nancy was leaving to play bridge. I had lunch and am off to a board meeting. We spend dinner together every night.

5:18 p.m.: Nancy is with her 99-year-old mother. She always gets back in time to have dinner on the table at 6:00 p.m. She is just a super lady. Everyone we've ever met tells me how lucky I am.

5:20 p.m.: Being married to Nancy makes me feel special. Nancy is very attractive and could have chosen someone who isn't fifteen years older than herself. She is the love of my life and is the most totally unaffected person I have ever met. What you see is what you get. After almost 23 years of marriage, I still want to do things to her body that would excite the both of us.

7:52 p.m.: We just had dinner. I think our marriage is strong. We get along, we can laugh, we talk to each other about our days, but we don't talk about our relationship.

9:17 p.m.: Here's a little history on how I feel accepting of Nancy's lack of interest in sex. Right after we moved to Florida fifteen years ago, Nancy was diagnosed with cancer, and had a hysterectomy. Since then our sexual activity dwindled to little, then nothing. We have had no intercourse in almost five years.

9:19 p.m.: After four or five years of no sex, I've become accustomed to it. The solution? Masturbation, of course. Infrequently, about once a month. I would much rather live with Nancy without sex than to live with anyone else with sex.

10:02 p.m.: Just spent the last two hours watching TV while Nancy watched TV and read. The usual way we happily spend most evenings.

SATURDAY

7:38 a.m.: Last night in bed it appeared to me that Nancy purposefully rolled over on her stomach so I couldn't touch her breasts.

8:17 a.m.: Just finished breakfast while Nancy did the crossword and Sudoku. I think Nancy sees the life she has now and is very thankful. I had a successful career at a tech company. She has more money now than she's ever had. Before we met, she found out her husband was having an affair and kicked him out of the house. She had $67, and he lost his job.

8:41 a.m.: I feel relieved because we no longer have a mortgage on our house. While I realize this may appear to have nothing to do with our relationship, it actually relieves the pressure and allows me to feel more relaxed, which I guess makes me more open to my sexual feelings.

10:24 a.m.: Nancy volunteered to help me put up a new flag on our community flagpole. It was nice to do something together.

5:27 p.m.: Off to cocktails and dinner for a friend's birthday. Going out is rare for us. We stay home for dinner together more than anyone we know.

10:08 p.m.: Just returned from dinner with two other couples. Mind wandered to how I would like to explore a "threesome." I have someone in mind. Nancy's sister is very attractive and she and Nancy would be great partners. I haven't tried it because Nancy would never agree to it, nor would her sister.

SUNDAY

8:35 a.m.: This morning, Nancy rolled over so we were face to face. I began exploring her body, but after a few minutes she brought that to an end with the statement, "I don't work anymore," and rolled away from me. I said, "You want to bet?" But she got up without a response.

9:16 a.m.: Sunday is the only day that Nancy does not do crossword and Sudoku, so I had a chance to ask her what she meant. Nancy said it all started with her hysterectomy and that her body aches all over and that penetration is painful and that she doesn't like oral sex. She also said that she feels sorry for me, but is satisfied to remember the great sex we had in the past. I said, "Are you sure?" She said she didn't have any sexual feeling anymore.

1:53 p.m.: Since today is Sunday both Nancy and I are spending the day at home. We have not talked further, so I guess it is what it is. I am going to accept that sex will never be in the cards for us ever again. It leaves me frustrated, but she's worth it.

4:57 p.m.: I met Nancy after my divorce from my first wife, whom I married before either of us were ready, and with whom I had many children and a 30-year marriage, until I had an affair. Call it midlife crisis. In the years between marriages, I was fortunate to have the company of a number of attractive female companions. I guess looks are important to me. When I met Nancy she fit the mold. She had a lot more going for her than just her looks.

5:00 p.m.: I belonged to a singles group that had a weekly house party. I wasn't looking for a relationship with a single mom with a teenage son. Two months later I met her again, took her to dinner, and we went dancing and later had sex. It was terrific so I thought I should see her again, which I did. We had a lot of sex. The best relationship I ever had was with her before we were married. We dated for two years but I really had a hard time convincing her to get married. I knew she was the one.

6:48 p.m.: Just finished dinner with Nancy. Told her about some of the things that I have been putting into the diary, but not everything.

I did not bring up anything sexual, as I believe that is a dead issue. I understand that after a hysterectomy it is not unusual for women to lose some, if not all, sexual desire. I have been reluctant to become more forceful in pursuing intercourse with Nancy because of this.

MONDAY

7:00 a.m.: Woke up thinking that my life is good—but without sex. That's the thing I think about the most. That I miss sex.

1:28 p.m.: Today is what I call a free day. Nothing scheduled. Nancy is out with her mom and shopping. Just finished lunch and about to run errands.

3:04 p.m.: I do worry about marital problems—just not my own. I just emailed my daughter, whose husband filed for divorce, and is requiring financial support. I also have a son who had an affair for a year before his wife found out. My other son has a serious illness and lost his wife. I'm helping in any way I can. Though with my kids, grandkids, and great-grandkids, there are many situations that affect my marriage. I have had to put my wife first and daughter second.

6:00 p.m.: Nancy's making dinner. She's fantastic. For my 80th birthday, all of my kids flew in without their spouses to surprise me, and Nancy organized it.

8:00 p.m.: Nancy and I are spending the evening the way we spend most: we choose to do different activities in different rooms. We don't force each other's preferences on the other. It leaves us free to enjoy whatever we like to do the most. I feel unpressured. I'm over eighty, so I take it one day at a time. Tomorrow is the first day of the rest of my life and this diary will help me make it better than the day before.

The Devout Grandma Whose Chemo Is Vastly Improving Her Marriage

78, Bainbridge Island, Washington

MONDAY

7:00 a.m.: I awoke at 5:30 this morning thinking "just two days until my last scheduled chemo." I am looking forward to getting stronger and hopefully healthier. It has been almost two years since my surgery for ovarian cancer.

10:14 a.m.: While Will watches *The Price Is Right*, we have sandwiches and soup. I was a widow for ten years when I met Will. My former husband was killed in a commuter crash, and I have five children from my first marriage. I didn't date at all in the whole ten years I was a widow. I just didn't even think about it. Will and I had condos in the same complex, and we met that way.

2:47 p.m.: Will waits on me if needed and cleans the house, and I just don't have any complaints. Most of the time we get along very well, but sometimes hurt feelings lead to shouting and tears. Earlier in our marriage, we did some fighting. Usually it was over trust issues. Or he'd tell me that I always had to be right, or he wanted to limit my contact with anybody other than his family and shared friends. It wasn't what I'd expected. Then when I got sick, he just couldn't have been nicer. I think he was feeling worthless, and now he feels he's really doing his part and doing a good job, so that's made him less insecure.

4:00 p.m.: I've been very close to his family, but he doesn't think much of my own, and they barely tolerate him. It's better than it was. Will had quite a temper and did a lot of yelling and screaming at me. My son finally came over and let him have it, and pointed out that I've never had difficulty getting along with anyone. Will has really transformed. The last four years have been very tranquil. I don't want to be disloyal to him at all, because he really is great and I appreciate him.

7:42 p.m.: Dinner. Kind of a relief not to have to prepare meals for six. We watch *Who Wants to Be a Millionaire?* and the news. We have chairs close to each other in the living room, and I read. Before we go to sleep, we pray together. We no longer sleep together, but we're still attracted to each other. We enjoy romantic encounters. That's a senior surprise!

TUESDAY

10:03 a.m.: At the library. We enjoy our volunteer jobs, sorting donated magazines for resale. I read a few books a week.

12:26 p.m.: Afternoon bridge at the senior center.

3:00 p.m.: Went to the hardware store for geraniums for our window boxes. A beautiful tradition for us the last 12 springs.

3:11 p.m.: I am an optimistic "pray-er" during the day. I pray for our family and for others who need prayer. So many have prayed for me since I was diagnosed. It has helped! I am thankful.

5:06 p.m.: Church. When Will and I first started going out together, he asked if he could go to church with me. I think as you get older you think more about your faith and what's going to happen. It seems more real to both of us. We talk about it a lot.

8:13 p.m.: Touching time. When I met Will, I really appreciated his wanting to have a sexual relationship. It was pretty good during the first five years. He was in his seventies. Now that he's 87, we just lie in bed together and please each other with a lot of petting and necking and kissing. We do it maybe once or twice a month. It's kind of like a date, and that's fine.

8:25 p.m.: It feels good to be hugged and to know that someone appreciates your body. It's surprising because he looks old, and I look worse than old—I'm bald. I figure if we still like each other this way, it's a real bonus.

WEDNESDAY

11:16 a.m.: My final chemo today, hopefully. My doctor is well regarded. We appreciate his frank and hopeful approach.

12:09 p.m.: I've had surgery about three times in two years. It has drastically changed the way I look. I look old now. I lost a lot of weight initially. It has changed just about everything. I needed a lot of help. He still thinks I look good, which makes me feel good even though I look in the mirror and know I don't. I'm feeling almost normal again.

2:00 p.m.: My first husband's birthday is coming up soon, and I usually get a phone call from all the children. We had been married over thirty years. I just miss him terribly, and my kids do, too.

8:35 p.m.: Will has a physical tomorrow morning. We have a list of concerns. We pray the Lord's Prayer together before we sleep. And the part where it says you forgive each other—we've decided that's a good thing to do.

THURSDAY

10:32 a.m.: Will wanted to cancel the doctor's appointment this morning because he is not well. I convinced him he needs to go. The doctor discovered atrial fibrillation and high blood pressure. He is at risk for a stroke. We will do whatever needs to be done.

10:54 a.m.: My body is reacting to the chemo I had on Wednesday. I'll feel better in three weeks. I am missing my kids and my grandchildren. We are all too busy.

12:00 p.m.: Just got terribly weak. Can't trust myself to walk from chair to kitchen.

4:13 p.m.: When we got married, intercourse was never spontaneous. We had to make an arrangement the morning of the day we were going to do it, and he had to think about it all day or something, and we'd do it at night. Viagra helped for a while, then it didn't help so much. Now we don't even try that.

4:42 p.m.: After I had a hysterectomy, I thought, I bet I won't even want to have intercourse. But I do have those feelings. One of the hardest things was a colostomy bag for nine months. It took a lot of care to be clean and not smell bad. I had another surgery to repair that. But I do miss intercourse. It's a surprise when I feel like I want it.

9:00 p.m.: I am so tired at night. But chemo hasn't been as bad as I thought it would be. I expected to be sick to my stomach all the time, and that didn't happen. Will has been wonderful.

FRIDAY

11:32 a.m.: Will's sons and their wives come to visit and discuss his health problems. They are a great comfort, and planted the geraniums.

2:53 p.m.: We are praying and we are thankful.

5:13 p.m.: When we got married our plan was to take care of each other as long as possible. We tell each other all the time that we love each other and we kiss a lot. He thanks me for everything that I do and I thank him, too. Now I feel like I'm getting better and he's having health problems and it's my turn.

5:45 p.m.: I expected I'd be with my first husband, of course, and enjoying my grandchildren. My grandchildren are pretty much grown up, and I haven't been a big part of any of their lives.

SATURDAY

9:22 a.m.: I'm weak and tired and my stomach is upset. My last blood test result came in the mail and it's not good. I need to be patient.

10:00 a.m.: Will is feeling better and his test results are good. We are glad we are home and we are coping. Our love is strong.

12:56 p.m.: I don't think of Will as my soul mate. I don't think there is just one person in the world whom you should marry. Will is so different from my late husband, but he's a good husband and I'm glad I married him. His first wife was closer to him than I am. He was married for 40 years before she got cancer, so it was a low blow to him to have another wife with cancer.

12:58 p.m.: As widows, we both know what it is like to be lonely.

7:00 p.m.: I don't think I've said anything here that his kids don't know about, except that their dad is still a sexy guy. That might surprise them.

Aspirers

Second and third marriages are commonly Aspirer relationships. It is because they have emerged from their first marriages with a clear list of dos and don'ts, which easily translate into the shared goals of the next relationship. "We both came out of abusive relationships, and decided that peace in the home is the most important thing, and peace between us even more important than that," writes The Self-Employed Family Man, who enjoys conditions that would drive many Lovers off a roof. "A good relationship isn't built on sex, nor is it held together by sex," he writes. And indeed, his is not.

The Self-Employed Family Man Who Fantasizes about an Uninterrupted Sleep Cycle

43, Atlanta, Georgia

SATURDAY

7:36 a.m.: Awake. Sleep hasn't been abundant recently. By "recently" I mean since my son was born in 2006. Since then there has always been a child in our bed. When my son got his own bed (still in our room), my daughter took over his spot between my wife and I. Don't get me wrong, I wouldn't change anything about my life.

10:23 a.m.: I spend the first part of my day fairly engaged in work, and the second part staving off sleep.

1:56 p.m.: So I have these hotel-room fantasies. Not of the prurient sort. No . . . I fantasize about an entire bed to myself, a dark room completely bereft of night-lights, and sleeping for a full and natural sleep cycle. I do this a couple of times a year. Last time I booked a third floor room facing the ocean. Before I went to sleep, I drew open the sliding door to the patio, so the waves would lull me asleep.

12:19 p.m.: What am I grappling with in terms of my wife? It's sort of a luxury to actually have the time to grapple. I don't, really.

7:20 p.m.: I must be the odd man out, because sex and relationships don't seem to compete for my time as much as everything else: the kids, the house, the dog. And these certainly aren't worries—they are just what happen to be in my immediate field.

10:13 p.m.: Whole family in the bed. I know you're hoping for some juicy sexual bits, but two kids under the age of three have made sex a nonoption. That part of our relationship is on hold.

SUNDAY

7:19 a.m.: The first thing I do in the morning is get on email, and it doesn't let up until dinner.

8:00 a.m.: My first marriage was a clusterfuck of anguish, and it ended far later than it should have, with me delightfully discovering that she was cheating. An easy way out. We both came out of abusive relationships and decided that peace in the home is the most important thing, and peace between us even more important than that. So it is very, very rare that we fight.

8:02 a.m.: As for my current wonderful wife, the circumstances of our meeting (online) were far from romantic. But our first kiss was one of irresistible magnetic attraction, and we had mutual friends. We relate to each other better than I imagined I could.

4:00 p.m.: Over at the parents' house for Mother's Day dinner. I guess when I was younger, the idea of some sort of constant sexual fulfillment was very important. It just doesn't occur to me even as much as it did five years ago. I don't feel like I'm missing out on anything.

9:36 p.m.: Chronic, machine-gun farting in a queen-size bed with my wife and two kids all snuggled together. Afraid I am going to kill them with methane. Whatever I ate over there did me in.

10:36 p.m.: Fantasizing about winning the lotto and sleeping money-worry free. That gets me hard.

MONDAY

9:22 a.m.: Coffee with my wife on the couch, next to the picture window facing out into the yard, just enjoying the portion of the morning before the kids wake up and our routines kick in.

10:01 a.m.: My wife also works from home. I have a portion of the house that allows me to cloister myself. We socialize with each other, and our children have the benefit of being raised around both parents.

12:14 p.m.: Masturbation. Interesting. Maybe I'll take it up. As things now stand, I don't really have the kind of time it takes to crank one out enjoyably. Instead, I eat drive-thru burgers while I run errands over lunch.

6:01 p.m.: Tired. It's 6:00 p.m. And I'm drinking coffee.

8:45 p.m.: I tend not to spend a lot of time even thinking about my marriage. When there's comfort and solidity in a relationship, it doesn't really occupy your mind. My relationship presents no problems. That doesn't mean we are never stressed, but it means that we are frank regarding the issues, and there is no pretense, no hierarchy, and little if any resentment.

9:01 p.m.: There are, of course, some areas that remain taboo. She has an adorable little muffin top that I just want to lightly squeeze. This is completely off-limits. We fellows tend to think that if it doesn't matter to us, it doesn't matter to them. Nope. A full day of silent treatment and some "spa cuisine" for dinner.

11:00 p.m.: The Mrs. and I tried to consummate—the kids were asleep, the mood was right, why not? In the middle, the baby cried. Nothing kills it like a screaming six-month-old.

TUESDAY

9:00 a.m.: Work. Summer is coming, and I'll be worried about meeting my financial obligations.

7:19 p.m.: Tonight she accidentally burned dinner, so I just picked up Chinese.

8:02 p.m.: Two things I have to remind myself: to not forget to let her know how much I love her, and to engage in adult conversation (no kiddie words).

8:30 p.m.: Talking over sleeping kids. When we were first married, we talked about all kinds of things. A bit of the vitality and casual conversation has fallen off.

WEDNESDAY

6:00 a.m.: Up early.

8:19 a.m.: A good relationship isn't built on sex, nor is it held together by sex. Sex isn't the only pleasure in the world, nor is it the only way we can express and explore intimacy with someone. Love is more complex than mere copulation, and when I am able to be intimate, it is made more special by its scarcity.

7:21 p.m.: Finishing up some work now. Sun is still shining, thinking about taking the family for a ride and getting some ice cream. Nothing warms the heart like a child dancing for joy with ice cream on their face.

11:00 p.m.: She decided it's time to have a little fun. Very, very nice. We may not get to it often, but when we do, it's a tectonic event.

Lovers

Lovers! Throwing caution to the wind since 1762. Our next diarist continues the now-familiar custom, abandoning all practicality to date a man who lives a multi-hour commute away, whom his daughter dislikes. His diary is a joy to read along with, as he discovers both the world of Lover relationships as well as gay sex, leading us through gay steam rooms in New York, the afterlife of the gay bathhouses that closed in the wake of the HIV epidemic.

The Gay Dad with a Hot New Boyfriend, and an Ex-Wife Who Hates His Guts

48, Union County, New Jersey

SUNDAY

10:15 a.m.: Woke up this morning with a raging hard-on thinking about my boyfriend, Ben. Stroked it for a while and tried calling him, but no answer. I want to save it for him, so I stopped. It's my 48th birthday today.

10:45 a.m.: Boyfriend sang me "Happy Birthday." I love him so much. We are always talking on the phone (first thing in the morning, last thing at night, many times in between). I'm playing basketball later today and we're bringing our kids to the game to meet each other. Won't have any private time for birthday sex.

10:46 a.m.: I'm also nervous. I was married for 25 years, but I came out several years ago and am now divorced. Ben and I are in a 1.5-year monogamous relationship, and he lives two hours away. My biggest worry is my two teen daughters, who live with me full-time, accepting my relationship with him.

12:15 p.m.: Ben called and his whole family (parents, son, sister) sang me "Happy Birthday." He has such a nice family.

4:00 p.m.: On my way into New York to see Ben, I sideswiped a bus and really scratched up my new car. Called Ben, and he helped me deal. He is always there for me.

4:15 p.m.: Got a Happy Birthday call from the first guy I was with. He was very important to me, but also impatient because he wanted to be with me. He even threatened to tell my wife and kids. He wants to get back with me. I've told him no directly, but he doesn't seem to care.

5:45 p.m.: Bite to eat with Ben, my daughter, and Ben's son, and they all watched me play basketball. Daughter seemed happy. We decided to not kiss or hold hands so that my daughter doesn't freak out. I usually do both with him, so it was weird.

7:30 p.m.: Daughter tells me that she had a great time, and likes him much better than my previous boyfriend. Phew! Now I just have to worry about my younger daughter, who feels anything I'm doing is against her mother, so she's torn up about it.

8:00 p.m.: Called Ben. He is so positive about my family taking time to get through this.

11:55 p.m.: Good-night conversation with Ben, but felt horny afterward and decided to masturbate to celebrate. I'm a size queen, so I fantasized about being on all fours and having a huge penis in my mouth and another huge penis in my ass at the same time. Fell asleep that way, and woke up later still holding my dick.

MONDAY

6:30 a.m.: Woke up hard thinking about Ben, but had to get it down quickly to wake up the kids.

8:00 a.m.: Spoke with Ben on the way to the doctor. I love that he has a child because he understands.

9:00 a.m.: Just had hemorrhoid surgery with rubber bands. Ouch, I guess I won't be bottoming for a while. It really hurts now but it's worth it. I love it when we have sex, but it takes him a while to come (which I really like), and sometimes it hurts if it goes too long— hopefully that won't be a problem anymore after I recover.

9:04 a.m.: Right now my favorite is when he puts me on my back and looks into my eyes. He gets on his knees and lifts up my ass to kind of "sit" on his lap while I'm lying on my back, and then puts my legs on his shoulders. He then rubs his cockhead along my ass and against my asshole. He gradually works his penis into my ass while he kisses me, pinches my nipples, and strokes my cock. At this point I'm in ecstasy and he can do whatever he wants. Sometimes he goes slow and easy, and then he switches to hard and fast, stretching his legs out and holding my hands down with his hands. It's really hot, and boy do we make a lot of noise. Then we hold each other and talk about how much we love each other.

12:30 p.m.: Thinking about the previous post, get really hard and jerk off. It was nice and slow: I got completely naked and played with my nipples and balls.

6:15 p.m.: Ran into my ex-wife while dropping off medications for her—it was the first time in a year. She's just out of rehab. She was civil, a first. I'm hoping we can again become coparents, because our daughters really need a mother who is clean and stable. I have both girls in Alateen, and brought them to several COLAGE (Children of Lesbians and Gays Everywhere) events.

11:21 p.m.: Good-night call. Love.

TUESDAY

10:00 a.m.: Sitting at my computer job, thinking about how much I can't wait until we can play without condoms. We are waiting six months—then we'll get tested and know that we are both clean. Ben lost some friends to AIDS.

12:03 p.m.: Call from the first guy I was with. We had such great sex. We were both versatile, so we never really knew where it was going to go, which I like much better than straight sex—in the end, you always know what's going to happen there.

4:00 p.m.: Surprised I saw my wife yesterday. I used to tell my wife she was the love of my life, until I realized she wasn't. I did not have any interest in guys through college, where we met. I can't put a time on when I started to question, but a few years ago I saw a therapist and joined a group for married men questioning their sexuality (there are lots of us out there). After some experimentation, I came to the obvious conclusion that I am gay. There's not much out there about coming out to your wife, so after lots of therapy, I told her, even though she's as a recovering addict. It explained some things in our marriage, and she seemed relieved, confessing to an on-off affair.

4:10 p.m.: As time went on, my wife became more upset. It was a huge blow to her. We'd had plans for our lives, and now we both had to start over again. Things got ugly—she slit my tires, she would pull up to my apartment and yell "fag." She eventually ended up in rehab. We are all hoping she can get her life back on track and be a good mother again. I pay some of her bills.

10:00 p.m.: I didn't get much time today to fantasize or even talk to Ben. I really miss him.

WEDNESDAY

7:30 a.m.: Text about how much he loves me.

8:00 am: Finally talked. I only see him one evening a week, and if we're lucky, a few weekend hours.

9:30 a.m.: On the way to work, just passed the sleazy hourly hotel that I've used a few times because I had no other place to go with Ben. So glad I don't need to do that anymore.

2:00 p.m.: At the health club, and see Tony. It's awkward. I've sucked a few guys in the steam room, and now I'm monogamous so I can't. One guy I sucked told me that "nobody would ever know." I wouldn't do that to Ben.

2:10 p.m.: My steam room actions before I met Ben weren't something I ever thought I'd do. I was very nervous at first. You learn pretty quickly which guys are interested. They give you a glance, and you look at them and "accidentally" touch your dick or lift your towel to wipe your face. There's also the more obvious getting hard under the towel and "pitching a tent." Once both are interested, you take off your towels and watch each other jerk off. I had a lot of mutual masturbation sessions—and one time a circle jerk with five guys. But I never touched anyone.

2:17 p.m.: After months of playing safe I was in the steam room, and Tony walked in and dropped his towel. I was newly out and had never played with one that big. I let him catch me checking him out, and took note of the time, so I could see him again. As expected, he came back the next day around the same time, so I smiled at him. He went into the bathroom, and I followed. He was at a urinal so I walked up next to him. He whipped out his huge penis and turned to face me so I dropped my shorts. We just watched each other jerk off and I was in awe of his much larger cock. We both came and left.

2:20 p.m.: Of course, I couldn't stop thinking about it. So the next week I looked at him while working out, and he followed me into the bathroom. This time when we dropped our shorts I had to touch it. I reached over and stroked it for a while. He stroked me, too. It was wonderful. I couldn't believe I got two hands around it.

2:23 p.m.: The following week I was in the shower waiting for him. I let him catch me looking, and sucked on my finger to let him know what I wanted. He came into the steam room after me. I decided I had to make my move, and said, "Can I suck your dick?" He dropped his towel. The first time that I tried, I gagged. Tried again, and this time got the whole huge penis down my throat. I couldn't breathe but I didn't care. It felt great. I took it down my throat a few times before he told me he was going to finish. They usually get thicker just when they climax and you can sometimes feel the load going through. I really like that. But I didn't know him so I was worried and backed off.

2:30 p.m.: Then one time after sucking him I asked if we could meet after work for him to have sex, and he said that he doesn't want to take it out of the gym. I was a little upset, but that's okay. I wonder if he's married. After that he didn't show a lot of interest. And now I'm monogamous.

2:45 p.m.: Tony said hi in the locker room. Every once in awhile I like to catch a peek of that huge cock and know that I sucked on it.

7:03 p.m.: Register for my high school class reunion. I brought my wife to the last reunion. It will be interesting to see the reactions to Ben.

8:00 p.m.: Jerked off. I imagine being with five guys at the same time: one in my ass, one in my mouth, one sucking me, and one in each hand, and then I have all of us climax at the same time.

8:02 p.m.: I'm upset that I can't see Ben. But we're focusing on integrating our lives, eventually moving in.

11:00 p.m.: Ben's giving me lots of good advice about what to tell the kids about their mother.

THURSDAY

6:30 a.m.: There is a Chinese medicine tradition called "morning prayer" that my boyfriend likes to do: he enters me, holds me, and looks into my eyes, only moving just enough to stay hard. Hopefully one day we can actually do it in the morning—we have yet to spend the night together.

10:00 a.m.: Going to go to the nude beach (gay section) today, but figure I should "clear it" with Ben. I actually spent a week at one several years ago.

2:30 p.m.: As expected, Ben trusts me to go. Though I don't go because I have too much work, and I'd rather go with him.

2:45 p.m.: Masturbate. I really liked it when Ben pinned me down by putting his knees on my shoulders, much like you do when you're a kid, and shoved his penis in my face and told me to suck him. I expect we'll be doing more bondage and toys (whips, handcuffs, etc.) soon. Ben's into it. He also shoved his ass in my face and told me to eat him—that stuff gets me really hard.

3:00 p.m.: Phone call with a basketball teammate about how he goes to the park to play with hot guys. It sounds exciting, but I don't know how he does it when he has a boyfriend.

9:00 p.m.: Spoke with Ben for an hour about our kids, spirituality, and other stuff. We could've used another few hours. I really want to see him in person.

6

ending

DISSONANCE, BREAKUPS, DEATH, AND OTHER MISHAPS

We are never so defenseless against suffering as when we love.

—Sigmund Freud

The Secret Behind Breakups

In the years before I began collecting diaries, I thought, based on a sample set of one (myself), that breakups were mysterious and somewhat unforeseeable, and therefore, often devastating. I've now had a front row seat to hundreds of breakups and come to see relationship turbulence as less of a death knell, and more of a natural progression of individuals' shifting priorities. Think "changing seasons" versus "emotional slaughter." When diarist couples fracture, I want to reach through the page and poke the diarist on the shoulder: "Hey, diarist! You two are adorable together, but your priorities are no longer aligned. Don't get too upset about this. It's common."

Instead, I'll tell you: the diaries are something of a looking glass for understanding relationship stability. Up to this point in the book, you've read 15 diarists in successful ongoing partnerships.

Ongoing because all 15 share two commonalities: (1) sexual and personality compatibility with their partner, and (2) the same shared relationship priorities. Barring extreme circumstances (third parties, health crises, etc.) those diarist couples will likely stay together for as long as both facts remain true. Because the diaries make one point clear: *When two compatible people like each other and want the exact same things on the same timeline, they very, very likely stay together.*

Not so for the three diarists ahead, who are all skidding on very thin ice. They once adored their partner, and are now navigating the deaths of their relationships. Invariably, at the heart of each struggling relationship is an issue of misaligned priorities. The two partners' priorities were once aligned—creating their shared relationship priorities—and now they're not. The demise of previously stable couples is rather foreseeable.

This understanding of breakups, by extension, defines what a relationship actually is: a connection built around 2–4 shared priorities, which shape the content of the couple's interactions. When those priorities no longer match, the whole relationship collapses. An analogy is useful: Imagine the two owners of a successful, tiny gourmet restaurant. Five years later, one partner loves the restaurant as it is, and the other wants to expand and franchise. No matter how well they get along, and how complementary their business skills are, conflict will ensue. Priorities are about resource allotment, which can't be compromised. The same priorities that pull us together force us apart.

The reverse is also true: periodically, I read diarists with partners who seem barely compatible: He's a nerdy engineer and she's a hippie doula, and their friends are confused. But their relationship works because they have the same priorities. The mainstream idea that "opposites attract" is incorrect: *priorities* attract. All sorts of surface daily sins can easily be brushed under the rug when two people, at their core, deeply want the exact same things.

Why are so many breakups so messy and painful? I am sure that you have, in your own life, watched in horror as two caring, logical people proceed to emotionally rip each other to shreds in a drawn out breakup. I can tell you that the most gut-wrenching breakups in the diaries take place when a diarist is very compatible with a partner—-perhaps they have similar social styles, or great conversations, or amazing sex, or the same outlook on life—but they have misaligned priorities. It's a gash at the core of the relationship. When breakups get ugly, it's often because of all the anger that flows from the unmet needs, creating detritus and hurt that obscures the gash. But the core issue is very simple. Their priorities don't line up.

Dissonance: How to Spot an Impending Breakup

The wording and cadence of diaries make it obvious which diaries are heading for Splitsville. A few tell-tale signs:

- *Should.* In the soon-to-fail relationships, there is often heavy use of the word "should," as in how things *should* be. Obviously, they're not.
- *Rhythm.* Sociologists find that people who are connected develop a rhythm to their movements, a kind of beat, very visible from across a restaurant. Or in a diary. As you read some diaries, you can feel the beat of the couple—or their dis-syncopation—through the page.
- *Dissonance.* Diaries often reveal dissonance between what the diarist is saying ("I love him") and doing ("I'm showing up 30 minutes late for dinner with him"). Psychologist Janice Kicolt-Glaser of Ohio State University has found similar dissonance in body chemistry: newlyweds will state contentment in their relationship, while releasing stress hormones into their bloodstream, indicating that a part of them is uneasy. That uneasiness is very visible in the diaries.

And, of course, misaligned priorities. What so confuses diarists caught in the crosshairs of an impending breakup is their ongoing sexual and personality compatibility. It's their *relationship* that's failing, not their chemistry. Over time, their lives are increasingly intertwined while their core priorities aren't getting met. Their relationship is like a high-rise building with no central support structure. The taller the skyscraper gets, the more disastrous its ultimate collapse can be.

Sexual compatibility, by the way, is not rare. Diarists are bonobo-like in their ability to have earth-shaking sex with many, many individuals. But successfully talk with, live with, sleep with, and align priorities with a partner? Not so many. All the sexual compatibility in the world doesn't help if a diarist wants one type of relationship, and a partner wants another. It just obscures the core difference.

Keep in mind that the diarists in this chapter are presenting their perception of their partners, which is biased. Men, in particular, can be less skilled at getting into a partner's mind and inferring their emotions. But their complaints? Those are always diarists' expressions of unmet needs. The louder the complaint, the more of a priority is to the diarist.

We head now to Washington, where The Secretary's many needs are going unheeded.

The Secretary with Three Children: Two Sons, and Her Boyfriend

50, Vancouver, WA

THURSDAY

8:36 a.m.: I woke up a couple of times last night having both hot flashes *and* cramps. Doesn't seem fair, does it? I have been afraid of going through menopause, worried that I will lose my libido in the process, which has created a sense of urgency within me to take advantage of my sexuality now.

11:06 a.m.: Sometimes I think I create drama with my personal relationships in order to make up for a boring work life, since my job category was downsized and I don't do much anymore. I'm now primarily a human security blanket for my manager.

5:45 p.m.: I get home and Gene is already upstairs in his office. Although the garage door opener rattles an announcement of my arrival, he claims that he "didn't know I was home." Why can't he simply act happy to see me when I get home? And dance?

8:00 p.m.: I mention my menopause concerns to Gene, and he says that, in his experience, post-menopausal women are "highly sexual and very reactive." That makes me feel somewhat relieved, I guess.

8:07 p.m.: Gene just told me I have a good body. The nice thing about being with a man who has such a vast knowledge of pornography is that when he tells you that, you believe him. Glad to still look good enough that my daughter's friends also make cougar/MILF comments about me.

FRIDAY

8:39 a.m.: Wake up watching Gene's naked butt as he gets into the shower. Nice view. I love it when he is the one to wake up first.

8:42 a.m.: I've been with Gene, 50, for two years. It's rocky. He only does what he wants, when he wants to, and doesn't take the needs of others into account very often. I think about ending it on a monthly, if not weekly, basis. But I am a serial monogamist. I was married for twenty years, then with another man for three.

10:41 a.m.: So much for actually getting anything done at work. Today is my son's college graduation. I am so proud of him for finally finishing.

8:47 p.m.: After the graduation dinner, we go out karaoking. My now-grown kids do a hilarious rendition of "In the Summertime." Gene didn't come to karaoke, but he has let me down in so many ways that this is not shocking. It was a wonderful night.

9:07 p.m.: My children feel that I can do better than Gene, and I am sure they are right. Their point is that my relationship has no benefits for me.

11:40 p.m.: Gene's asleep. I guess one of the things that bugs me the most is that he seems so (relatively) uninterested in sex since we have become a couple. This month, we have had sex only six or seven times. Sure, we both had the flu so that took up a few days, but that's a huge dropoff.

SATURDAY

9:49 a.m.: I am picking up my niece and Gene's teenage daughter. Gene's daughters are actually part of the reason that it is difficult for

me to break up with him. They are nice girls who lack a strong paren-
tal role model.

10:00 p.m.: Tonight should have turned into intimacy, but he was
nervous/anxious/whatever about me secretively taking the time to
write this. It's bugging him.

10:05 p.m.: He made a joke that I have started an online romance
on a dating site. Part of the reason I don't trust him is that during the
summer we first met, Gene was having sex with three different women
(me included) at the same time. Once I saw his calendar, I realized he
had sex over 24 times that August. That has gotta be an impressive
statistic for a 50-year-old man.

10:15 p.m.: I had no idea that it was so easy for men to have multiple partners. Gene took advantage of my trusting nature, and this
continues to plague our relationship. I know that during our summer
weekends together, he was sending quick texts/emails to the other
women.

SUNDAY

8:17 a.m.: Lack of physical intimacy makes us both antsy, and we
had better do something about it soon

12:15 p.m.: I quit sending daily emails to Gene about three weeks
ago. I am trying to pull away from him, and be more independent.
When I first met him, we exchanged emails throughout workdays.
These days, I can't tell if it's some sort of power play, or if he really
doesn't think about me at all during the day.

1:00 p.m.: I'm realizing I will probably never be in love with someone again the way that I was with my first husband. Perhaps I will be
able to find the type of man that I want to spend the rest of my life
with, but the majority are like Gene, selfserving and lazy. As the saying
goes, "Why buy the whole pig, when all I want is a little sausage?"

7:58 p.m.: No, Gene has *not* sent me an email today, and it's not
like he is too busy, fer crissakes. Thank God for Facebook, or I would
go completely insane.

8:03 p.m.: I really hate this kind of double life that I am living. On the
one hand, I am positioning things for my imminent breakup with Gene,
and on the other hand, I am signing up for a class with his daughter.

10:15 p.m.: We just argued on a subject so incredibly trivial (he didn't like the way that I got into bed) that it clearly indicates he has something bigger going on. He is probably getting fired tomorrow, and I think he's worried whether I will kick him out of my house once he is unemployed again.

10:20 p.m.: What spins me up about Gene potentially losing his job is that this is falling back into the pattern of last summer, when he was at home, bored, all day long. Not a good situation for someone who has had a problem with porn addiction. I don't like the idea of him masturbating while I am at work, and I also don't like the idea of coming home to a man who is all hot-n-bothered from looking at naked women all day long. To me, masturbation is just slightly north of pathetic, anyway.

MONDAY

8:30 a.m.: Last night was the first night ever that Gene and I didn't snuggle at all for the entire night. No kiss. No nothing. Really, if there is going to be no physical contact at all, I would rather sleep by myself. It's too much effort to lay there *not touching*.

11:11 a.m.: Just sent a long, thoughtfully written email to Gene, addressing some sticky points. Talking to him in person is difficult because he overrides me.

12:11 p.m.: Call Gene. He says that, no, he hasn't read my email yet, but no, he wasn't busy with other things, either.

7:39 p.m.: Meeting up with Gene and his two daughters to have dinner together. Oddly enough, he seems more excited to see me than normal. Don't know if it's because of my email, or because he wants to put on a good appearance for his kids.

10:30 p.m.: Gene ended up talking with his ex and daughters tonight, which is fine, but he gave no indication ahead of time that he was going to take his time coming home. So I assumed there would be no sex happening and got in the bathtub, which he hates because he likes how I smell at the end of the day. Just as I was getting in the tub, he got home, and ended up getting in the tub with me, which was just exactly what it would have taken, at that point, to stop me from being annoyed with him.

11:45 p.m.: Sex. A very romantic and satisfying evening after all.

TUESDAY

8:25 a.m.: Wow, Gene is bubbly today. It turns out that he did end up getting fired yesterday, so he is happy. He hated his job, and would rather be on unemployment.

8:36 a.m.: I realize that I am on a downhill slide with Gene. He refuses to accept normal adult responsibilities. Once I have broken up with Gene, I will never again put myself in such a vulnerable financial position. I also know that I will never give up hope of finding someone who, while not perfect, is perfect for me.

9:53 a.m.: Email from Gene, requesting to continue our online Scrabble game. We have been playing Scrabble for a year, but I would rather not anymore, because he cheats. He doesn't know I know.

9:54 a.m.: If someone cheats while playing a game, won't they also cheat in other things as well?

10:01 a.m.: How long will it be before Gene gets caught up with his porn addiction again like last summer? The threat is always there, looming on the horizon. I have read that intelligent men are more likely to become addicted to porn, because of their greater ability to fantasize. He acknowledges that his addiction played a large part in the destruction of his marriage.

11:20 a.m.: Although there's a little too much drama sometimes, I am basically very happy with my life. Sure, I would rather be settled in a last-love relationship with the man of my dreams, but it's not like I am missing out on life in the meantime.

· · · · · · · · · · · · · · · · **Diary Insight** · · · · · · · · · · · · · · · ·

The majority of the diarists in this book are regular porn viewers, particularly in this chapter. The next diarist realizes that he's carried the notions of pornography into his bedroom. Which is the equivalent of watching a Hollywood movie and trying to reenact its plot points with your family. Not going to happen. Each of the next two diarists are realizing that their use of pornography is a reflection of their *own* relationships to sex and has nothing to do with their wives.

· ·

The Marketing Guy Realizing That He Views His Wife as a Porn Star

37, Washington, D.C.

MONDAY

9:10 a.m.: Carpool lane at nursery school, dropping off all three kids. A woman I don't know just started talking to me. My thoughts gravitate toward wondering if she wants an affair. Why?

10:15 p.m.: Working in the home office. My wife is an amazing person and she's pretty damn hot. She has an awesome butt. She wears thongs a lot, which I now see primarily in the laundry. But we're pretty emotionally distant right now, so physical connection isn't even on the table.

10:56 a.m.: Sometimes I fantasize that my wife will just come in and give me a blow job.

10:57 a.m.: In a bajillion years, that will never happen. I know her.

10:58 a.m.: I also secretly harbor fantasies that my wife would have anal sex. I've had it before, and it's pretty good. She would never do it. The fact that I am thinking about this when there's no prospects of sex on the horizon just shows you how much I am kidding myself. Not that there should be any prospects, since I was a total asshole for a long time. Still.

5:25 p.m.: Really trying to grow out of a guy who thought about sex as a physical act for self-gratification and looked at his wife as only an object. For a long time, I treated her like a hole for my personal pleasure. I feel like I just need to take this one day at a time. The longer I go, the less desperate I feel, like I can get to a place where it's not all about the physical. Sometimes I feel empowered.

6:05 a.m.: My sister-in-law is over, playing with the kids. It makes me uncomfortable that I find one of my wife's sisters to be sexually attractive. I'd never do anything about it, but it's awkward. And I'm someone who doesn't get awkward very often.

6:59 p.m.: All I said was, "The shirt is poofy around the side." My innocuous comments are all so misinterpreted. Men think about intention. ("I can help you look better.") Women think about impact. ("You made me feel fat.")

7:00 p.m.: I tend to only hear the criticism, not the praise. So it feels like most days that I am just a colossal fuck up. The walking on eggshells makes me sad, because it's not the "happily ever after" vision I was sold. I don't want it to be this way.

7:57 p.m.: I think I am compensating for the lack of intimacy by overeating. Not so healthy.

10:45 p.m.: So! My wife just told me that after two months, she's ready to give sex another try. A large portion of her willingness, apparently, is due to the fact that she fears that if I "don't get it," I'll "explode in anger." (She thinks I'm often angry. I think I'm just intense.) I worry that a marital sexual relationship based upon her fear of my emotional explosion is not a strong one.

11:45 p.m.: I've come to the realization that I've had a lot of sex, but I'm not really certain that I've actually "made love." That makes me feel a bit empty and makes me wonder if I can actually ever do it.

TUESDAY

6:08 a.m.: I used to go out of my way to sneak a peek at my wife as she was dressing. The teenage boy in me was thrilled. Now I've begun averting my eyes (not always successfully). If I can do that, I may be able to begin to stop viewing her first and foremost as a sexual object, right?

6:10 a.m.: Averting eyes. I have to say, my wife is just really, really hot. I just want to jump her bones. Of course, that's what got me into this mess.

10:37 a.m.: Over the years, I have become much more of a person of faith. I recently found *Garden of Peace,* written by a rabbi. He basically says, "Look, your wife—with all of her irrationality—is a vehicle that God uses to help you achieve self-perfection." Let's put aside the potential misogyny. I've found it a really valuable coping strategy. Now I simply think "Okay, you are a messenger from God. There's something that I need to look at in myself and you are just reflecting that. What is it? How can I improve?"

10:42 a.m.: Normally, I would take a porn break. But in the two months since my wife and I had sex, a few things have happened. At first, I decided that I'd cope with any sexual tension in as positive a way as possible. No thoughts of other women, no porn, no whacking off. If I felt the urge, I'd do sit-ups. It worked.

10:44 a.m.: My wife, however, was worried I'd "explode." She said, "You should masturbate. It's normal." She reads a lot of health stuff on the Internet. So, I did. The first time in seven weeks, it felt great. Then, I enjoyed it less and less. I am trying to find the courage and strength to view sex and ejaculation as part of a larger context. I'm like a sex addict in detox. I haven't been able to explain that one to her yet.

10:47 a.m.: I think my first exposure to porn was when I was 10. On some issues, I think feminists are nuts, but they are right on in the way porn warps men's minds in how they view women. You don't even realize it until it's too late (if ever). Instead of learning to love my wife physically, I sort of viewed her as someone I could turn into a porn star. That was a stupid idea.

10:49 a.m.: The porn exposure thing also made me value numbers of sexual experiences, devoid of true feeling. I don't know how many sexual partners most people have, but I had a "goal" of double digits, which I have achieved. I think this is what aging is. Realizing how stupid and lame you were when you were younger. I fear for my son.

2:34 p.m.: Work call with gay colleague. I wonder if gay men are more sexually satisfied. You know—similar drive, more willingness. I probably will never ask. It's not the kind of thing you post on Facebook.

5:25 p.m.: So my wife tells me again that she thinks she is ready to have sex tonight. I'm a guy and, of course, getting laid is the best. However, I realize intellectually, that this is a lot more than that. And that makes me scared. This is a pivotal moment in our lives. If it's a bad experience for her, we go down one path. If it's good, we go down another one. I really feel self-doubt as to whether I can make it good for her.

5:27 p.m.: I think she's doing this for reasons that are about me, not her. I think she views it as something she just has to tolerate. Not the ideal.

11:09 p.m.: Sex! Well, it took us two months, but my wife and I had sex tonight.

11:15 p.m.: When we were in the middle of it, it felt like it was a huge, pivotal life moment. I knew that we were beginning the healing process and hopefully reestablishing trust. It's going to be a long road ahead and, I hope that like a broken bone, it's stronger when it heals.

11:18 p.m.: I'd be lying if I said it didn't feel good. I'd also be lying if I said that I wasn't nervous. I was. Very. Still, I think it worked out okay.

WEDNESDAY

8:32 a.m.: Outside school, and three dads just turned to stare at the same passing mom. We all saw each other looking, and everyone smiled and kept moving.

8:33 a.m.: Just FYI ladies, this is a special "male-bonding" moment that occurs when guys who don't know each other share a similar view. It's like, "Yeah, bro, you were right to turn your head for her!" You both know that you saw it and "won."

12:00 p.m.: One of my wife's biggest issues is that, usually, after I get "it" (sex), I'm no longer interested in being nice the next day. So today I've doubled down on doing just that, and being helpful. I think it's working.

12:10 p.m.: I do realize that I've taken my wife's love for granted and not reciprocated. It's made me realize what a selfish ass I've been.

6:00 p.m.: On the phone with my mom. My wife finds her to be very imposing and interfering. She tolerates my dad, whom she respects, but finds him borderline arrogant.

11:10 p.m.: Wife's asleep. From now on, sex, instead of just a physical act for my own pleasure, has taken on a more symbolic role. Do I still really like it? What kind of stupid question is that? Of course I do, but I am slowly beginning to see the role that it must have within a marriage. ***

Why Multi-Decade Relationships Last

Why would two people who really like each other and fulfill each other's needs split? They don't. And hopefully, their needs shift in tandem over time. The Minister Who Just Discovered Himself has not been so lucky. His is among the most compelling diaries in the book, a man whose needs have shifted drastically in the thirty years since his marriage, creating oceans between him and his wife. "More than anything I want intimacy," he writes. "I long for the touch of my skin on another being's, being unselfconsciously naked, open and giving." A visual listing of their priorities is helpful:

Her + His Relationship Priorities Circa 1979
- Religious partnership
- Security of a life partner
- Daily companionship

His Relationship Priorities Today
- Spiritual soulmate connection
- Sexual exploration and fulfillment

Hers never changed. Note that there's *no overlap,* meaning they each want a completely different relationship. He deems his marriage a failure, but he is not looking at his long marriage on its own terms: he and his wife have created precisely what they set out to attain, a family of faith. This is often the case with diarists—they build exactly what they intend. And then they change their minds.

The Minister Who Just Discovered Himself, Porn

56, Western North Carolina

TUESDAY

12:00 p.m.: Very busy week, in a different city each day. Just finished addressing a conflict in a family. A central part of my work is creating relationships that are open and honest without being destructive. Many people wouldn't identify what I do as healing, but they would look back later and realize that their life was changed through work that I did.

3:00 p.m.: Meeting of a group of businessmen. Part of the discussion was about how to avoid lust. The very fact that we were talking about lust was creating an environment to be lustful. It was on our minds already. You can't fight it. Coming from a faithful background, there are all these prohibitions against sex outside the marriage, against masturbation, against pornography. And there's no counterbalance that says, "To replace that drive or inhibition that you're having, do _____." So it's really an inadequate ideology, as far as I'm concerned.

8:30 p.m.: Home. I'm tired. My wife of 28 years went to bed before me. We don't sleep together. We've been celibate for over a decade. There is a level of incompatibility that was easier to gloss over when we were first married, but no longer. Do I want it this way? No. Am I responsible for this situation? Yes. Do I have any control of it? Very little.

10:31 p.m.: Most pornography is boring. It is all so self-consciously sexual. I'm a minister. I'm a traditional person. Most people don't even know that I think about these things. In my world, there is no one to talk to. The majority of people I know are prudish or fearful.

10:40 p.m.: I checked out a punk-girl website of artsy nude photos. Those are the girls I want to know. The most interesting thing I saw is a gallery of photos called Fight Club, like the movie, except girls. What's interesting is their lack of self-consciousness. Where does that come from? That ability to be naked from the waist up, with no sense of self-consciousness about it? Maybe it's all a show, but I don't think it is.

1:00 a.m.: I sleep in my grown son's room. I sleep naked when I'm there. I won't sleep naked with my wife, because she's very private. She brought that with her into the marriage. I've probably had sex with my wife a dozen times in 28 years, and neither of us had had sex with anyone before our wedding night, when I was 28.

WEDNESDAY

8:30 a.m.: Tried to express my true feelings about my father's recent sudden passing, and ended up in an argument with my wife. I don't blame her. Until I was probably 50, I was a very unemotional, detached person. It affected her to the point where she's not interested in me. What has given me strength has been my faith in God, in Jesus Christ.

12:00 p.m.: Meeting six new clients at lunch. Two are women, mid-30s. They are attractive and confident, don't flirt, and look you square in the eye. I like them. Impressed with who they are. When there's some chemistry, I ask myself, "Is this someone that I'd be willing to lose my marriage over?" I have not yet met that person.

1:34 p.m.: Drive two hours to two meetings. Sometimes being by myself traveling gives me time to gain perspective. A few years ago I took a job that kept me away much of the time. I became very lonely, and realized why my wife was angry at me, and hated me for my inattention to her and lack of support in the ways she needed it. It was a revelation of monumental proportions. I was transformed. That's when I began to sleep without clothes on. I masturbated a lot. But unfortunately that was just my experience. I came home, and everyone else was the same.

6:30 p.m.: Community event. Nice people. The key is finding out both what they want to achieve and where their pain is. New opportunities emerge as a result.

9:30 p.m.: Too tired to drive home. Check into a hotel. Typically when I get to a hotel room, all my clothes come off and I get in the bed. And occasionally I will masturbate. It's actually to remove the outside world from my conscious brain. I find a great deal of freedom. It's a release of pressure from the outside.

9:45 p.m.: The first time I masturbated was on a trip like this, probably 20 years ago. Purely out of scientific interest. I heard a side conversation about it, and thought, "I've never done this. I don't even know what this is all about." So I bought *The Joy of Sex*, which describes how to do it. And I was away on a trip by myself, and I did it for the first time. It was enjoyable. And I didn't do it frequently at that point, but it became something I turned to when I realized that my wife and I were sexually incompatible. It's frequent now. Could be every day for two weeks, could be once or twice per week. Stress has a lot to do with that.

11:00 p.m.: Beer and dinner in the hotel restaurant. Sat at the bar, just wanted to be alone. So tired. Watched three 30-something women flirt with the bartender. He was gracious, but not amused. For men, sex is escape. A return to the womb to find relief from the stress of life. For women it is relational, and for men it is often not. For everyone, it's a feedback mechanism to validate their value as a person.

11:58 p.m.: Long couple of days. Met many new people. Sleep.

THURSDAY

7:30 a.m.: Take a long walk. Streets are empty. Quiet is nice. No distractions. I'm finding it really interesting to articulate my relational thoughts here, because the media provides language to use—and it's not what you really want to say.

10:00 a.m.: Driving to a luncheon. In seminary, I saw that many people's spiritual development was simply using God as a vehicle for staying focused on their own self and development. I see it all the time.

6:00 p.m.: Dinner with family. Good time for catching up. My (mostly grown) kids play Wii after dinner. My son is on his second long-term relationship, and while we wish he would choose people who were more challenging to him—in the right way—we're glad he has those relationships. I do talk about relationships with the kids, but we don't talk about sex. No one does.

7:00 p.m.: Men's group. I meet with ten guys from church twice a month. We catch each other up on what's going on in our lives, and look at some scripture. Occasionally, one of the guys will remark about his wife. What is clear is that all of us are not well-connected to our wives. And it isn't one of those things where one person is clearly to blame. It's much more complicated than that.

8:15 p.m.: Realizing that I have never heard anyone in the group talk about this stuff. I never hear that. Never. And I don't think it's a social stigma that causes it. It's not a stigma. I think it's more of an internal emotional dilemma we have.

9:00 p.m.: I wish that my wife would go have an affair. It would be so freeing for her. Because she is so emotionally constrained. I surely love her. I just don't know how to love her in a way that removes the barriers that exist between us.

4:00 a.m.: I often sleep for three hours, then wake for a bit around now. The thought has begun to occur to me that I may never have sex again. I ask myself whether I could live another forty years that way. The jury is still out on that question.

FRIDAY

7:00 a.m.: Drive three hours to a meeting. Talk on the phone with my wife about family schedules. You know, I'm a very linear thinker. And for the first twenty years of our marriage, I wasn't comfortable in the emotional aspects of relationships. Most romantic situations aren't linear. There's no game plan, no logical progression. You start in the middle and you're thrown in a direction. I didn't know what to do with that. It all happens on an emotional plane, and I had no way of being emotional.

10:00 a.m.: Spending the day facilitating a board retreat. I'm running the meeting, so I have to stay on topic. Not much time to reflect on interpersonal relationships.

12:00 p.m.: I want to say something about boards. People join them with their own experiences that they're trying to protect. They have a really narrow and limited view of what the organization is about, so I spend a lot of time establishing a context so they can think more broadly. The romantic lesson here is that it's not always about you. Which is frequently the media's depiction of romance—that it's about what you can get out of people. It's not.

10:00 p.m.: Guesthouse. I didn't call my wife, sleep, or masturbate. There was a TV in the lounge, and I watched a baseball game.

SATURDAY

9:00 a.m.: Back with the board to do a wrap up. There is a woman here and it's clear that she has an issue, some hurt or pain. I see that a lot. And sometimes I envision interviewing them where the two of us are naked. And part of this is telling a woman what I see that I want to affirm. Because I get the impression that women don't get affirmation in the right way—that they're not affirmed for who they are on the inside, but for how they look on the outside. And it really comes out of a desire to help the relationships of women. I know that because I don't have one with my wife.

2:30 p.m.: Finished up the board meeting, driving home. I wonder what it would be like at a naturist resort. To be naked with a bunch of strangers seems really awkward to me. It really isn't the nakedness, but whether there is any social recognition of the penises and vaginas, or are they treated as not there. I wonder about that.

4:00 p.m.: Got home. The family was watching a movie. I went into the bedroom to change clothes. Masturbated. And returned to watch with them.

10:00 p.m.: My wife's already asleep. In my work, I talk with people about transition points. That point comes when things that worked well in the past no longer do. I feel I'm at that transition point. More than anything, I want intimacy. I end this diary longing for the touch of my skin on another being's, being unselfconsciously naked, open and giving.

Breakups

For every newly-in-love high in the diaries, there is a corresponding emotional ditch. (*Shhhhh*, don't tell the diarists in chapter 3.) And in the years before I began editing the diaries, I approached the specter of relationship endings with the same nuance as the diarists: pleasant, abject denial. Each new relationship was like moving into a new home: I overlooked the loud neighbors and crack in the ceiling, unpacked the 50th box, and promised myself that I'd be there for a while.

Nothing knocks the legs out of that logic like a summer spent reading thousands of diaries, each of which discuss a handful of past and current lovers. That's, oh, 1,500 diarists talking about upward of 6,000 lovers. The unavoidable deduction is that all relationships—every single one—comes to an end, one way or another. Some stick around for fifty years. Some don't. It's a cycle. And both diarists ahead thought, until quite recently, that they would break the curve.

I tell you this because it's quite liberating to be freed of the Myth of Happily Ever After. Although the option of clinging to someone else makes life seem less overwhelming and scary, it's also limiting. It shuts the door to all of the wonderful possibilities that most diarists in this book are embarking on.

What startled me most, though, was the stack of diaries from which I've drawn this section: relationship refugees whose minds are still in a relationship that, to the outside, ceased to exist months or years ago. Their minds are still firmly Partnered, still perceiving themselves in terms of their partner, and thinking as if they are in a relationship. Yet they are clearly single. It's a state of mind all its own, and I call them semi-solo.

How is this possible? Call it an unfortunate trick of the mind: The brain's long-term-attachment wiring is primitive, with the evolutionary aim of encouraging couples to stay together long enough to rear a young child. It whirls along happily when the partner sticks around, pumping the brain full of mood-enhancing hormones. And if the partner suddenly disappears . . . it's not good. The brain's love mechanisms are the equivalent of a well-designed sports car for which no one bothered to design brakes. It keeps on revving and revving, drawing on an empty tank. The diarist's only option is to let the car coast until it rolls to a stop. "Just like someone going through chemical withdrawal, a lover becomes anxious and unable to concentrate in the absence of the partner," writes Tara Parker-Pope in *For Better or For Worse.* "Even a small dose of affection—a phone call or a text message—gives them their 'fix' and calms them, at least for a while." The brain chemistry of heartbreak mimics both obsessive-compulsive disorder (plummeting serotonin levels) and addiction (active dopamine receptors). This is why The Lovesick Texan Who Mistakenly Dumped His Girlfriend feels like he's "dying." His personal hell makes for one of the most familiar diaries in this book. His brain is essentially in a full-blown mental illness, the standard human response to a split, fueled by little boosts each time he hears from his ex-girlfriend through the day. He can't think of anything else, from the moment he awakes and awaits her first text message: "This is the hardest part of the day, while she's asleep, or whatever. . . . It's hours and hours of waiting." Notes, emails; and voicemails temporarily paralyze both diarists ahead.

Relationships that take place in one's own mind are rarely written about, mostly because they sound crazy, and because those who survive the experience want to forget it promptly. But it's normal. Really normal. I see semi-solo diaries all the time, most commonly identifiable by internal monologue conversations with their ex, and a diarist whose mind is convinced that all would be well if things could just go back to the way they used to be. Every braking car has a timeframe all its own. Some roll to a stop swiftly; others peskily roll on long past the end of the road that the physical world sees. In the meantime, the diarist has a hard time focusing on work or anything else—that job promotion has little meaning from the Darwinian perspective. (Fisher suggests, by the way, that rerouting this obsessive thinking is best done by essentially mimicking addiction treatment: toss out all traces of the person, and stop communication, weaning the brain.)

Bad judgment abounds in these diaries. The Pining Mother's friends are baffled that years after the split, she's still in love with her cad of an ex. It's brain chemistry, not logic. Fisher put 15 brokenhearted research subjects under MRI scans, and showed them photos of their lost loves. Their dopamine systems, which manage addiction and pleasure, began firing; the areas of the brain that manage anger, irrational behavior and risk, and obsessive-compulsive urges also lit up; hers and other studies have connected heartbreak to physical pain.[1] Yes, all of that forehead banging and acting out is *scientifically visible*.

What these diaries don't show is the health impact of these splits. The end of relationships hits people hard. Divorcées and widows of all ages suffer an immediate decline in health from which they never recover, including 20 percent more chronic health problems—a dip so marked and abrupt that some researchers hypothesize that losing a partner might spur a chromosome to switch on. Widows go on to have lower amounts of sex than any other demographic, 11 times per year, due to a combination of age and lack of a partner.

Male and female diarists experience the end of relationships differently. Men take the ends of relationships more harshly, and are 2.5 times more likely to kill themselves following a breakup—they, in fact, fall in love faster and harder than women as well. "There's nice data that men do feel passion as much as women," says Fisher. But they are also better compartmentalizers. "They may be very involved in that difficult breakfast conversation, but then they get to work and can put that aside." It's because when testosterone washes over the developing brain in the womb, few neural links are left between the front and back of the brain. Estrogen links the two brain regions.

"Men seem to be better at tunnel vision, just focusing on what's going on now. But if you prompt them, you can focus them," says Fisher.

Three things to look for in the diaries ahead:

- Diarists almost universally describe their recently lost relationship as "unique" and "special." I call this the tyranny of the special. It loses its charm after a couple hundred sightings. The truth is that falling in love is often a predictable mix of compatible biochemistry and aligned priorities. What the duo created may have been special, but not that fact that their particular quirks attracted each other.

- Breakups tend to be more painful when the diarist experiences emotional pain very differently than the partner. Both diarists ahead qualify: their partner inadvertently sets off a string of negative, looping thoughts that can last days, and wanders away—because the same behavior would have no effect on them. Diarists who understand the way their ex feels pain are able to, in many ways, prevent this.

- Diarists tend to take roughly half the length of a relationship to get completely over the relationship—no pangs or pining thoughts—up to five years. The Mother Pining for her Jackass Husband is pining because after 20 years of partnership, her brain is effectively wired to do so. There are no hard rules. "It was like a veil," writes The Grandmother Who Is Perfectly Happy Alone, in chapter 2, of life without her husband of 40 years. "I was trying to look through a veil, and it took [5 years] for the veil to lift. And now I'm off and flying."

What always strikes me about the diaries of the recently split or widowed, more than the details of their stories, is how, as a culture, we are horrific at dealing with death of any sort. The diarists are unprepared for it, and are surrounded by well-intentioned friends who don't know how to support them beyond the first two weeks cooking and providing tissues. These diarists suffer for a long time, and often end up, emotionally speaking, as animals on the tracks, despite their best efforts otherwise. More than anything, these diaries are reminders that the end of any significant relationship is more of a life passage than anything else. There should be a party. Or a dissolution ceremony. With or without the ex. It's a noble idea: a gathering of friends to acknowledge the death, and move on. Relationships are a cycle, and the diarists in this chapter are about to flow into something new.

The Lovesick Texan Who Is a Hot Mess without the Girlfriend He Mistakenly Dumped

38, Dallas, Texas

THURSDAY

7:19 a.m.: I wake up, and have a good 15 seconds before I remember the mess I've created with Samantha.

8:00 a.m.: Nine months ago I thought I would eventually die alone and unloved, but then I met someone who was crazy about me, and I was crazy about her. I've been single a long time, and when things got complicated and hard I wasn't sure I could even be in a relationship, so I accidentally broke up with her. I now realize that all I want is to be with her. We've been talking about trying again, but she has been seeing someone new for the past month.

9:17 a.m.: This is the hardest part of the day, while she's asleep, or whatever, and I haven't heard from her. Just a few months ago, when we were together, I woke every morning with a text from her. Now it's hours and hours of waiting.

11:19 a.m.: She texts me to say that the guy she is seeing is meeting her at a burlesque show on Saturday, but she wishes I was, because it would mean more to me. She emoticons a sad face.

3:07 p.m.: I try to keep my mind busy with other things: work, my newsreader, a biography. It sometimes works for whole minutes.

3:20 p.m.: I've recently read through every email we sent over the six months we were together. I've been trying to figure out where things went wrong, and where I could have done things differently.

4:51 p.m.: The Savage Lovecast can't even save me this time. Okay, it saved me a little bit.

7:26 p.m.: It's been a little over nine months since I met her, and a little over three since I broke up with her. It's been almost five weeks since we last had sex, almost three since we last kissed, and almost two since she told me she's with someone else. It's been, like, twenty years since I was in high school. Hell if I can tell the difference.

7:38 p.m.: I've been crazy about her since the night we met, but I broke up with her one stupid night. It just wasn't working, and neither of us had any answers about how to fix it. She keeps asking why it will be different now. I've given her a dozen reasons, but I'm still looking for the magic words.

10:50 p.m.: I decide to go to the bar, to take my mind off things. Before I've had half a drink, Samantha texts to say she is thinking of moving to Austin. I should've started with shots.

FRIDAY

9:46 a.m.: Austin isn't a deal breaker for me. We've talked about her moving away for grad school, and her hope is that if we got back together, we would stay together even though she's in another city. But this isn't grad school, and we aren't together, and I'm worried that she is trying to run away from her problems.

11:34 a.m.: Samantha texts me a close up of her breasts in rhinestone pasties. "Aren't they pretty?" she asks. She might be trying to kill me.

1:11 p.m.: I email K, someone I've mildly made out with a few times since Samantha, and invite her to happy hour. I think romantic interest has fizzled for both of us, but we usually have fun.

7:24 p.m.: Never hear from K. Work late and go to the bar anyway. It's almost all gay guys tonight. Not even the cute lesbians-who-might-be-thirteen-year-old-skater boys.

7:27 p.m.: I get kissed on the cheek a dozen times by the Banana Republic guy whose name I can't remember. It's the most action I've gotten in weeks.

8:11 p.m.: My family is fundamentalist Christian, and the less they know, the better we get along. I was still very religious when I first became sexually active at 20. The poor girl. We would park and fondle and go down on each other, then afterward I would feel guilty and tell her we could never do that again, and then we would the next night. She had been raped a few years before. I told her how sorry I was and how awful that was. Then I told her, real helpful like, that in order to heal from it, that one day she would have to forgive him. I actually said that to her.

8:41 p.m.: You should know that I dated two more women, and depending on your definition, I was still a virgin. The last one was on top of me, and if I'd raised my hips I would have been inside her. She rolled off of me and said, "I can't." I felt really screwed up after those relationships, and I stopped dating for five years. I just wanted to get myself together emotionally. I stopped believing in God. I drank alcohol. I worked. And when I lived in New York, I couldn't get a date to save my life. By 30, I was ready to date again, dying to fuck for the first time. I met a librarian. We got along great, and on our third date she came home with me. She had three orgasms while I was going down on her. Then I told her I was a virgin and she was okay with it. And it was great.

9:16 p.m.: I lost my virginity listening to Björk. And not the Sugarcubes. Vespertine.

11:51 p.m.: Totally irrational, but I get a little angry when people text me who aren't her.

SATURDAY

9:38 a.m.: Text Samantha good morning. She used to wish that I would be the first to text occasionally. She texts back that she hates today.

1:13 p.m.: I'm convinced that she likes me more than she likes him, that I'm better for her, that she'll be happier. I think she knows this too. But in the meantime there's all this anxious waiting.

1:19 p.m.: She calls to say hi. I don't talk about relationships or feelings or anything like that. You're welcome.

2:48 p.m.: In my mind, a relationship looks like this: a couple sitting in a coffee shop reading, or on a patio sipping Bloody Marys, or holding hands walking down the street. It's nice and calm and content. But that's only how it looks from the outside, isn't it? From the inside, it's messy and restless and sort of scary.

7:06 p.m.: I'm bad at dating. Rarely do I see anyone for more than a couple of months, so I don't know how to be in a real relationship. As much as I wanted to be with Samantha, I wasn't looking at things the right way. She needed more from me than I thought I was willing to give. If I could have held on a little longer I would've gotten there. Now I'm there alone.

7:25 p.m.: My theory is that by the sixth month of dating someone, you should know whether or not there is a future. I've stopped seeing two other people around the six month mark, and the theory seemed sound. Though I did continue having occasional sex with one of them for another . . . Jesus, 5 years. What the hell is wrong with me? Anyway, the theory seemed sound until now.

7:45 p.m.: But I broke up with her impulsively, without thinking. Because we weren't talking, because she was making herself sick with insecurity. Why will it be different now? Because my heart and my head finally want the same thing.

9:11 p.m.: I rarely masturbate for pleasure lately, but use it as a way to hold back my libido. I usually do it once in the morning, and if I have time, again at night. The morning I found out that Samantha was in a new relationship, I masturbated 4 times. Tonight I do it before showering and meeting my best friend for a drink.

SUNDAY

12:21 p.m.: It's been a rough morning, knowing she was with him last night, and imagining that she still is. I get called into work. It doesn't help.

12:53 p.m.: I'm surprised by how heartbroken I am. I didn't think I would ever feel like this. I feel the urge to self-destruct.

2:12 p.m.: Samantha calls. I act like I'm not dying.

2:42 p.m.: We talk for a half hour, and she says she'd like to see me today. We're interrupted when her ex-husband calls about their child.

3:38 p.m.: Pick her up to go to lunch. She answers the door in cutoff jeans and a tank top, her hair in a bandana, and no makeup. She looks gorgeous, and I tell her so.

4:05 p.m.: We talk about all the difficulties she's having coping. Money, parenting, school.

7:08 p.m.: We decide to go for a drink, but I drive aimlessly instead. She says his name for the first time. She tells me about him, the good and the bad. There is a lot of bad. There is so much bad I'm shocked she is with him. Debts and drugs and warrants. He is insanely possessive and hot tempered. On the plus side, he makes her feel really special.

8:55 p.m.: On a bar patio, sipping vodka. I want to take her home and watch her undress. I want to feel her skin. I feel shitty about this.

11:30 p.m.: She says she almost kissed me. I say I really want to, that I really want to do more than kiss her, but I'm afraid that if I do that and we get back together, that it will make her suspect I'm cheating on her. I've never cheated or been cheated on. She has, and she gets suspicious easily because of it. She says I'm right, and we stick with just the emotional cheating.

11:45 p.m.: We stand up to go inside the bar. I stop her and ask if she has a feeling about what's going to happen. She says she does, and leans against me. I put my arm around her. Things feel right again. We talk for hours.

3:35 a.m.: Samantha's boyfriend is waiting when I drop her off. He asks who the hell I am. I haven't touched her all day, so I feel comfortable. He says, "It's not worth it," and leaves. Then he comes back and I tell her I can't leave her there. She says it would be best if I left.

3:53 a.m.: I circle by her apartment. They are still outside. She says he wouldn't hurt her, but I'm not convinced.

4:10 a.m.: She texts that she left her keys in my car, but that I shouldn't come by.

MONDAY

8:56 a.m.: I make it to work on time, but exhausted. I text her to ask if she is okay. She says yes.

3:22 p.m.: K emails to ask how happy hour was on Friday. I think briefly about telling her I might be getting back together with my ex, but don't.

7:09 p.m.: The Banana Republic guy definitely has a crush on me. He gives me an invitation to an event tomorrow at his store and makes me promise to come. Then he gives me his phone number and says we should hang out. Hoping this is one of those ignore-it-and-it-will-go-away situations.

7:26 p.m.: Samantha texts and asks if I think I could get sweet-rough with her in bed. I thought that I already was. A flurry of dirty texts.

7:59 p.m.: I'm pretty sure she's masturbating on the other end of her text messages. I'm so turned on I can't stand up.

2:26 a.m.: Samantha tells me she knows she has to break up with him, but she has feelings for him, and doesn't want to break his heart.

TUESDAY

8:27 a.m.: I worry that she feels stronger about him than she does about me, or that she is going to remember it that way once she breaks up with him. I hope distraction will be on my side this time.

1:38 p.m.: I eat a sandwich in the Gayborhood, and on my way out I see some flyers and the word "apostolic" catches my eye. "Apostolic-Pentecostal-Welcoming-Affirming of All." I grew up Pentecostal. They are certainly not affirming of all.

3:54 p.m.: When people think that I'm gay, I tell them they are probably just picking up on the repression and self-hatred.

6:20 p.m.: With the librarian, and everyone I've dated since then, I've explained my situation, and said that because of that I want us both to be able to see other people. No one has ever said no to that. Samantha is the first person I've agreed to be exclusive with since I was 23.

6:45 p.m.: Dinner with a couple. Friends. I tell them everything.

8:00 p.m.: Samantha calls. She misses me and wants to see me, wants me to come stay with her, but she hasn't broken up with her boyfriend yet.

12:57 a.m.: My friends want to go to the gay bar. I give in. This is what naked men smell like? I cower against the bar. Bored and sleepy, go out to friend's car to nap until they're done.

WEDNESDAY

10:00 a.m.: Samantha texts to ask about my night, and to meet her for lunch.

2:06 p.m.: With Samantha at a restaurant. She's beautiful, always so beautiful. As we eat and talk, I feel her leg against mine under the table. I love this girl.

3:30 p.m.: Hug goodbye. A long hug. I whisper in her ear that I miss her. She doesn't say anything. She gets in her car and I tell her to drive safe. She doesn't say anything. I feel nauseous, forever. I love this girl, but she scares me.

4:13 p.m.: I'm not acting like myself. I'd probably feel a lot better if I'd dragged her into a closet and fucked her until she couldn't see straight.

4:15 p.m.: Samantha texts me to "just be yourself, the person who makes me go weak." She is right.

9:32 p.m.: Drinking with a female friend. She wants to talk about Samantha, but I don't want to. I know she wants to protect me, but I want to protect Samantha. It gets tense at times. I know she can be irrational, and that the problems aren't gone, but I want to be with her.

10:05 p.m.: I was really happy being single and uncommitted before. But now that I've met Samantha, single and uncommitted don't seem like happy alternatives anymore. I want to be with Samantha.

The Mother Pining for Her Jackass Husband Who Left Her for Another Woman

52, Western Massachusetts

FRIDAY

8:35 a.m.: Woke up to a sweet, loving voicemail from Russell, the man I recently broke it off with, letting me know that he's sent me a letter. Now I miss him. I have been protecting myself a little from those feelings. I'm not sure how glad I am that he called.

8:38 a.m.: I'm away on a writing retreat, while my husband has the kids. We're separated, getting divorced. Since getting separated, I was in an intensely loving and sexual relationship with a man named Russell, though I am now alone, and sometimes it is excruciating.

9:29 a.m.: Just did a guided meditation about what gets in the way of direct experience of your life. I thought about how I want to be more receptive to the warmth of the relationships that I already have.

2:30 p.m.: Went to the beach and ran along the shore. It was completely deserted and so I laid topless in the sun and felt somehow very complete.

5:30 p.m.: I miss my children, the affection, the physical contact. I feel untouched.

6:52 p.m.: Thinking about how free I am. I don't have to respond to someone, I don't have to be flexible. I have control over my own space. I usually feel more lonely, so I am grateful for this feeling at the moment.

SATURDAY

9:56 a.m.: Last night I dreamed about buying Nancy Friday's My Secret Garden. They didn't have it in stock but said they could order it for me and all of a sudden I was embarrassed to be speaking about it with the saleswoman. I am so interested in other women's sexual fantasies—I've never talked about it with my friends, and wonder where people go in their minds.

11:32 a.m.: Heard the voice of my ex-husband on the answering machine, telling me something about the kids. A wave of missing him hit me so hard. He said he wasn't feeling well, heartburn. I couldn't miss the irony in his word choice.

11:33 a.m.: Most people don't understand why I still have such deep and loving feelings for him. All I can say is that it doesn't have to make sense.

11:34 a.m.: My main introduction to cell phones and email was betrayal, the form my ex-husband used for many years to communicate with his lover. He had a code name for his girlfriend's number that looked like his office. Once, in a particularly desperate moment, I checked his cell phone and found more than 10 a day to that one number. In over twenty years, I hadn't even opened his underwear drawer or datebook. But I didn't have the nerve to check the number. Of course, part of me didn't want to know: it couldn't be true.

3:24 p.m.: Returned to the deserted spot on the sand where I could lie topless. It is an amazing and arousing sensation to actually feel the wind on my nipples. I didn't want to leave.

5:00 p.m.: A fantasy I had today running on the beach: A man was also running, in the other direction, and he looked at me and then turned to look again. He looked like an actor I couldn't quite place, not an attractive one. And I remembered that I'd hoped this week away maybe I'd meet someone and have wild sex with him.

6:00 p.m.: On the beach I was reading Adam Phillip's book *On Kindness*, and he quotes Freud as saying, "We are never so defenseless against suffering as when we love." I feel that speaks so much to the inherent vulnerability that I've felt now for so many years in losing the relationship I wanted for the rest of my life.

8:17 p.m.: I spoke with a friend tonight who asked if I was lonely being away. I said it surprised me that I mostly wasn't, that I've been very content alone and very happy not having conversations besides those with my children.

9:23 p.m.: It's my last night here, and as I anticipate going home, I can feel all the relationships I'm returning to, my children, my ex-husband, the daily contact with him, the heartache. I've realized how much being in relation with others can take me away from myself, my desires, my attention to my own needs. So to celebrate I sat outside in the dark with the moon out and smoked a cigarette, which I'd brought here on purpose. Haven't had one in years. It was delicious.

10:00 p.m.: Making efforts to push away images of my ex-husband and his girlfriend together being sexual. It is those images that make it hard for me to fall asleep.

SUNDAY

9:08 a.m.: I woke up crying this morning. It feels so hard to be returning to my divorced life: the glimpses into my ex-husband's new life, the effort it takes to allow my children to have their own relationship with a new woman.

9:15 a.m.: One part that's so hard is how sexually drawn to him I still feel, and how torturing it is to imagine him with someone else. In the months before he left, we had the most passionate, intimate, vulnerable sex of our long marriage, and I told him then that I didn't ever want to regret having that experience with him. And yet now the memories of it make me ache, literally.

10:00 a.m.: This morning I meditate outside and the sun is so strong on me that I take my shirt off, just like at the beach, and I'm so aroused by the feeling of being half-naked outside that I go back inside and lie on the unmade bed and touch myself until I feel intense pleasure. It feels like a gift to have moved into this headspace from where I was just an hour ago.

10:01 a.m.: Sometimes I wonder about being sexual with a woman, as women's bodies are very arousing for me to look at and imagine. But when I think of actually touching another woman, I don't feel as interested. I do wish that when I was younger I'd explored having a relationship with another woman.

12:40 p.m.: One of the things I miss in my relationship with Russell is the spaciousness of the time around sex. How we could spend hours talking after. That was so new to me, to spend so many hours in bed after we'd been so opened up to each other through sex. I've never felt so vulnerable with anyone. I miss that deeply, finding new places in myself with him.

8:41 p.m.: Profound sadness. Because I so didn't want my children to go through the wrenching separation, as I did when I was a teenager. And I realize that I have been so devoted to wanting my marriage to work and being available to my children and husband that I overlooked the limitations of what I have control over in my life. I somehow believed that I could make this work too.

9:14 p.m.: Home. Back in the midst of laundry, dishes, bedtimes, homework, schedules, and negotiations—and although I'm aware all of these domestic details are part of a foundation that I sometimes take deep pleasure in, I wait for bedtime, just to have moments alone, to come back to myself. It's worth the subsequent lack of sleep.

10:00 p.m.: Reading Russell's letter to me. Am reminded of the deep connection we do have, where time melts away and both of us find a way to truly be there. I ended it because I couldn't bear the pressure to be more available to someone who was so unavailable in so many organizational ways. Yet he was more available emotionally than any man I've been involved with.

MONDAY

6:49 a.m.: I wake up and wonder about calling Russell.

7:01 p.m.: Coming home from a long day of picking up and dropping off kids, work, and then picking up and dropping again. I'm struck by how crowded it is to return to daily life.

8:01 p.m.: Run into a friend in the store parking lot. She separated around the time I did, and is still in the relationship she left her husband for. She tells me that her ex-husband is thinking about dating someone I know, and she asks me if I'm still dating Russell. I say no, I feel better on my own. But then I drive away, and I feel suddenly lonely and unpartnered, out doing all the tedious errands alone. I wasn't feeling alone before I talked with her.

8:04 p.m.: I worry that I will spend the rest of my days alone. I keep this a secret because it feels humiliating, and I worry there's something about me that makes me so hard to live with, and yet I know I have so much to give.

10:16 p.m.: I just want the day to end now. I want to wake up and feel different tomorrow.

11:01 p.m.: I just wish I had someone here who wouldn't talk to me, who wouldn't want anything from me, who would willingly and lovingly massage my back, my head, my ears, my neck, my feet, until I fell asleep.

TUESDAY

8:35 a.m.: In my mind, replaying the greatest hits of Russell's disorganization: He never washes his clothes or sheets, and the food in his fridge has been rotting for months. He is late for everything, and getting out of the house can take 30 minutes with returns to retrieve everything. He stays up all night, sleeps sometimes, never eats or exercises regularly, and falls asleep during most movies and plays. Then there was the time he couldn't find his car keys and kept me waiting for an hour outside a restaurant on my birthday in the freezing cold and never called—and then was annoyed that I was upset.

8:52 a.m.: Wondering if anyone will ever find me attractive again. And also, just as importantly, if I'll ever find another man attractive again.

8:54 a.m.: It was an amazing experience to discover in my relationship with Russell that, even in my fifties, I am so deeply desired and
admired. And to feel that urgency in desire. This has been a surprise and
a delight, and I remember thinking at the beginning of our relationship
"How will I ever get any work done?" as I felt so consumed with desire.

9:10 a.m.: Email from Russell. I'm drawn into his beautiful way of
writing, the way he still cares deeply about me even though we're not
seeing each other, and I'm reminded of what it is to have someone in
your life who can picture your day, the piles on your desk, who knows
the foods that you cook. It's a kind of intimacy that I deeply crave.

10:12 a.m.: Just got my period in full force with painful cramps,
and I'm shocked at times how strong my periods can still be in my 50s,
how bright red and vivid the blood. It seems a sign of persistence.

8:35 p.m.: Russell called just to see how I am. I'm struck by how
well he knows me, how he jokes with me in a way no one else has been
able to. I lean into his voice and relax. But I also know that I am more
relaxed by not being affected by his chaos and disorganization, by not
trying to figure out how to fit a relationship into my life right now.

9:19 p.m.: Even though I've been clear that I don't want a regular
relationship with Russell, he wants to go away with me for a weekend:
swim together, eat good meals, see a movie, spend hours in bed making
love and talking. He says it will be good for me. He even tells me it's
good for my children that I am loved like this. I'm not sure what to do.

11:35 p.m.: The other day I fell in my mud room, after tripping on
a shoe. And it was the strangest thing to lie there, alone in my house,
and think that no one in the world knew I fell. Or even would know
unless I told them. Which I never did. I realize at this time in my life
how much more meaning those small moments in life have when
shared. For me, this is part of intimacy.

WEDNESDAY

10:53 a.m.: Coming from meeting with my two closest friends. I'm
entering into a long day of work without a lot of space for these kinds of
thoughts, so I'll just say that I feel buoyed up right now by all my friendships, the depths of them, how remaining connected to them sustains
me. I need to remember this when I am feeling abandoned and alone.

10:57 a.m.: I feel so triggered by some contacts with my ex-husband. I feel he's still lying to me; it is such a familiar feeling, the sense he's leaving out details. It can send me into such a dark place, with all the memories of the years I was being betrayed and was made to feel like I was the crazy one.

8:32 p.m.: I've been surprised by how full of sexual desire I have become as I've gotten older. Even before I got separated, I felt growing desire, an ability to feel more comfortable with my own sexuality and to talk more about sex.

9:42 p.m.: Since taking off my wedding ring, I now notice how many people wear them. I never looked before. I was always amazed when friends would tell me that they noticed. I think of myself as a perceptive person, but wedding rings were never what I was drawn toward. But now, now that I am divorced, it is a whole other thing. I see Obama's wedding ring flash gold in photographs. And my own ring finger hurts sometimes, it truly does. It still feels empty, as if it's missing something.

11:38 p.m.: It is a hard thing to admit to still being in love with my ex-husband, despite all that he has done that has made me feel dishonored and disrespected. And it feels harder to admit it knowing that I am an intelligent woman with many resources. And yet I feel so drawn back to him, to the life we built together, to the depth of our history, to our relationship around our children, to the unrealized aspects of our life together that I was genuinely looking forward to developing. I can't really say this to anyone. No one gets it. I think he does, actually. He knows. It doesn't change anything, but he knows. ***

Death

Next time you're in a room full of couples, announce, "Hey, guess what? All of your relationships are going to end!" Everyone will hate you. Quickly. Because for most diarists, particularly those under 40, denial about the fact that their partner might die lives at the core of their continuing efforts.

The two diaries ahead are quite different from the previous three, because in a breakup, it's the relationship that dies; in these, the partner dies. And a partner's death doesn't necessarily mean the relationship is over. Why should it end? Relationships are a state of mind, and for many widows, the relationship continues on long, long after the death. The Well-Adjusted Widow talks to her dead partner regularly, her mind's relationship engine still humming along two years later. And it's not sad. It's just real. There's a great divide between diarists who have been widowed and everyone else. Loss is only a taboo subject among those who haven't experienced it.

Masturbation is always fraught for diarists grappling with loss—it's hard enough when the ex is still alive. (The Lovesick Texan just described it as a necessary evil "to hold back his libido.") The Well-Adjusted Widow weighs whether the inevitable fantasy of her husband is worth the post-orgasm tears. The Successful Consultant dodges this by imaging her previous, well-endowed boyfriend.

Much can be learned from the widow diaries, beginning with their laments. They don't crave conversation, sex, or even family. The Well-Adjusted Widow craves being held, as do most widow diarists. In chapter 7, The Newly Widowed Player craves the walks he used to take with his wife. These diarists are appreciative of the little things: the hugs, the little outings. Cuddling is not something that partnered people tend to think all that much about. They are finely attuned to what truly matters in relationships.

We begin in Chicago, with a diarist who meets her unexpected loss with ample good humor.

The Well-Adjusted Widow Still Carrying on a Relationship with Him

53, Suburban Chicago, Illinois

THURSDAY

6:23 a.m.: Lying in bed pondering a new relationship. Not with a man but with a dog. A new rescue. Should I save a greyhound or get another labradoodle? Torn.

12:00 p.m.: You could say that my last relationship ended suddenly, when the aorta of Chad's heart split apart, his pericardium filled with blood, and his heart could no longer beat. I came home to Christian, our teenage neighbor, running up to my car to tell me that Chad was down, to finding Chad blue and lying in the driveway. CPR from Christian, me, and then the emergency techs did not work. His body was taken away less than three hours later. However, Chad and I still have a relationship. He still loves me and I still love him.

12:02 a.m.: It occurs to me that my strongest relationship is with a dead man.

12:10 p.m.: Sad. Not sad to be alone. Sad that I have gone from 4 (Chad + Chad's daughter + Chad's dog Nemo + me) to 3 (Chad + Nemo + me) to 2 (Nemo + me) to 1 (me).

12:27 p.m.: Email from the labradoodle lady: "I will have Kleenex waiting for you if needed when you pick your puppy up." Need Kleenex now.

3:48 p.m.: Just got back from a walk. The 20-something women in the apartment complex don't make eye contact with me. They know there's no good reason for a fifty-ish woman to move into an apartment by herself. I am the ghost of Christmas future.

5:34 p.m.: Was cc'd on an email due to an address typo: "I have your mobile and will ball you at 7:48 if you are not on the line!!" That is the closest I have come to nonsolo sex in a long time. I haven't been interested in anyone else since Chad died two years ago, and I'm not looking for anyone. A woman friend kissed me on the top of my head last week and that's been my only kiss.

9:11 p.m.: Headed to bed. This is when I hold my stuffed toy coyote and talk to it as if it were Chad. If I didn't talk to the coyote, who would I talk to?

FRIDAY

7:40 a.m.: Realized that a labradoodle puppy requires a whole heart. Can I do that again? A greyhound represents a lower-level commitment. I can open my home and just a little bit of my heart.

8:37 a.m.: I don't fantasize about sex. I remember sex.

10:13 a.m.: Saw a client who hugged me. Business hugs are the only kind of hugs I get these days. Better than no hugs at all.

11:48 a.m.: Looking in my recipe box for my banana bread recipe. Don't find it. Instead find Chad's Recipe for Love: Take one part Chad, one part Kat, peal all clothes off to bare skin. Some memories make me sad. This one makes me happy.

5:45 p.m.: I'm glad my hair is growing back. Much of it fell out after Chad died. This makes me think of Chad's curly blond hair—not on his head—which makes me think of how exquisitely perfectly his shaft was attached in the thicket. So I'm not dead. I'm just lusting after a dead man.

6:04 p.m.: I decided to get the labradoodle. I am building a life without Chad. New condo. New dog. I miss Chad, but I'm not done living yet and I've told him so. And I told him that when I get to the other side, he better be there waiting for me.

6:05 p.m.: In the past two years, I was able to bury Chad, give away Nemo, sell the house, move back to Chicago, and keep my act together enough to support myself through it all. I am proud.

7:03 p.m.: I am going to watch a chick flick rom-com tonight. Don't know how this will go. Mostly I've been sticking to documentaries. Testing the waters.

7:08 p.m.: I'm thinking about relationship expectations. My first expectation was to get married and have kids. Then my expectation was that the man I loved would love me back. But he wanted to marry me, not love me. (How many people go on their honeymoon and have sex once?) Then my expectation was to be on my own and feel safe. Then it became a hope that maybe sometime before I die, I would love a man who would love me back. Then it became a joy and surprise that a man (Chad) did love me and I did love him back.

7:10 p.m.: Then life got very simple: All I wanted was to live my life in such a way that I could spend as much time with Chad as possible. My unspoken expectation was 20–30 years together, and that he would die first, because I expect to live into my 90s.

7:11 p.m.: I only got 5 years, and more love than I believe most people get in a lifetime. I am glad for that, thankful that I know what it is like to be with a man who adores me day after day, who errone-ously believes that men fall at my feet when I walk into work, who in the morning says, "Sweet Baby, you are so beautiful." I didn't expect it to end so soon, but I never expected it to happen in the first place. So in the balance, my life is better than expected.

9:15 p.m.: Thinking about the night I got out of the office late and I told Chad a joke. He asked where I had heard it. I said I heard it online. He said, "This is what you were doing when we could have been together?"

SATURDAY

5:00 a.m.: Awake. Deciding whether or not to masturbate—plea-sure followed by the pain of missing Chad, usually ending in tears.

5:10 a.m.: Started, and then got up to go to the bathroom. Back to bed and back to sleep.

6:52 a.m.: Awake again, thinking about maybe masturbating but a hot flash starts, and that ends that.

8:10 a.m.: I wonder if I'll ever want to have sex again with anyone but Chad. So far it doesn't look like it. The idea of sex with someone else grosses me out.

8:15 a.m.: I met Chad through a friend and I hired him to build a fence and pour a concrete parking pad. Based on how he treated me, how he interacted with his workers and my neighbor, and not having had sex in 5 years, I propositioned him. He said yes. He thought I was beautiful and he treated me tenderly and he told me the truth and he loved me and I loved him back.

1:30 p.m.: More young women in the apartment parking lot who don't look at me. They don't know I'd rather be me than them.

4:36 p.m.: Figuring out what I want to do tonight. Last night I watched the rom-com kissing scenes very closely. I am trying to feel what it feels like to be kissed.

SUNDAY

7:23 a.m.: Lying in bed, thinking about my day. I play with my pubic hair with my left hand. It feels good. New discovery—some-thing sort of sexual that doesn't remind me of Chad.

11:00 a.m.: Therapy. She asked if interest in men feels like betraying Chad. I said no, I'm just not interested. But I do miss male companionship and holding hands. We decided that maybe I need a gay friend.

5:10 p.m.: Thinking about Christian. After Chad died, I asked him how he was doing. He said, "Kind of grossed out."

"About what?"

"I kissed a dead guy."

MONDAY

7:50 a.m.: Sitting at a work conference with my new friend Bridget, talking about a first date she's having tonight. We agree that the featured speaker would be good to have sex with, or marry, or both.

8:38 a.m.: He has been talking for less than a minute when Bridget says, looking at his left hand, "He's married. All the good ones are."

"No, they're not."

"They're not?"

"No, they're not. I promise."

"I'm just waiting for him to get divorced."

That's exactly what you want. The first marriage is a screw up: He's marrying his mother and you're marrying your father because you're trying to work out old stuff. What you want is to be #2. Number two is good.

7:43 p.m.: I am sexually attracted to two men! They are on the cover of *Vanity Fair* magazine, soccer players in very tight briefs. Photo men with paper skin.

8:28 p.m.: A dish of Java Mashup ice cream. The most physically pleasurable part of today.

8:33 p.m.: Email from Bridget: "We are all living in this dating purgatory, somewhere between the fleeting memories of bliss and the burning reality of its absence."

TUESDAY

11:30 a.m.: Work conference. If it weren't for work, I would have been home when Chad died, instead of finding him in the last few minutes of his life. Thinking about it, I'm actually glad at the way it worked out. It would have been worse to see him keel over. It helped to have the neighbor's warning first.

11:45 a.m.: Bridget's online guy didn't meet her last night. We declare him a fucker.

3:23 p.m.: Riding the escalator, I pass a woman on a cell phone. She is leaning my way. "I love you and miss you," she says. There is no one I call to tell them I miss them. There is no one missing me.

10:56 p.m.: It is past my bedtime, I have a lot of work tomorrow, and I have just written about Chad and sometimes thinking about Chad makes me smile and sometimes it makes me cry. Tonight it is making me cry because I miss him. If he came back magically for a day or even a minute all I would want to do is lie down next to him and hold him and have him hold me. That's all. That's everything.

WEDNESDAY

10:52 a.m.: I was interviewed last week for an article on surviving the loss of a spouse. Heard this morning that they can't use me because we weren't legally married. I feel illegitimate.

11:30 a.m.: The people at the deli counter I frequent are the people I know best in town, along with the people in the leasing office at the apartment building. I'm feeling a little lonely right now.

9:10 p.m.: Had dinner with a friend, Marianne. Marianne is going home to her husband and I am going home to just me. And that's okay—I like just me. And I learned the hard way a decade ago that I would rather be with just me than somebody just to be with somebody.

10:11 p.m.: How do I feel? I stand alone. But not really alone, I have friends and I have Chad flapping his wings. I would have preferred if Chad had hung around a bit longer but I'm learning how to live like this. And I'm looking forward to seeing him again. So I feel both good and sad. Glad to be alive. Miss being loved and touched. Not ready to go yet.

The Successful Consultant Whose New Soul Mate Is Dying

63, Northern Florida

SATURDAY

6:38 a.m.: This is a favorite time of day. Alan is asleep and breathing well, sleeping soundly—a good night. Now I do a little yoga, breakfast, and a walk before the world wakes up.

6:44 a.m.: Replying to an email about Alan's stay in intensive care this past week. It puzzles us—and even annoys us a bit—when people call us "gallant" and "inspiring." For heaven's sake, if the choices are moping or going out for barbecue with an oxygen tank, what would you pick?

9:00 a.m.: A successful shower today for him. We figured out a way to wrap his arm so the catheter line stays dry.

11:43 a.m.: Alan is off to the Mayo Clinic for another IV with his brother, so I am just doing the endless futzing that keeps things running. On a lark, because we know life is shorter than we think, we're asking a fellow we just met to come cook gumbo for us and a few other new friends on Sunday. He'll be by in a few minutes to check out the kitchen. Alan's idea.

12:48 p.m.: Finished filing, and throwing out old files. When living with the uncertainty of Alan's health, I hang on to the joy of orderliness. The reason for the end of our relationship is pretty darn easy to foresee. Death. The how and the when are the only mysteries. And I am afraid of the shape of those two unknowns. I am hopeful that his mind stays clear.

1:45 p.m.: You could say that there are more than two people in our relationship. We have a terminal disease as our constant companion. The trick is to be aware of her and her power, while remembering the stunning power and joy of love and the everyday. It's not always easy. There's a fine line between thriving in the moment and denial. We are clear-eyed and grateful.

3:25 p.m.: Heading out to a chick flick with friends. Alan is home from Mayo, and exhausted. His blood pressure is low, but a nap will help. And his brother is here—so not much to worry about.

5:33 p.m.: Alan is cooking. While getting his IV, he saw a recipe for stewed chicken on the Food Network, and had to cook it. Hard to believe he was in the intensive care unit on Monday—but he just keeps chugging.

5:55 p.m.: I am immensely grateful for the last two years. We met three years ago and felt not only instant love, but comfort and familiarity. On our first weekend together, we told the waiter that it was our 40th anniversary—and it could have been. They served us desserts on the house, for which we felt guilty. I moved in two weeks later. Three months later, he became ill, with a then-undiagnosed condition. I never blinked. It never occurred to me to leave, and it still doesn't. This has been the richest time of my life, and although we haven't had sexual relations in a year or so, in the affection and cuddling (when he's not hooked up to something) we are still like kittens.

7:09 p.m.: I am deeply happy with my personal life, despite the clear knowledge that there is not much time left. There will be a big hole when he leaves. Air sucked out of the room and house and universe. I spent a night at home when he was in the hospital last week, and the space was so empty, as if all the air had been drawn out, leaving in its place stale vapors.

10:00 p.m.: Our intimate life is warm and affectionate, but sex is not a part of it any more. He's just too weak. At first it seemed like a big loss, but now not so much. We both know the end is very near, and so the importance of what's no longer possible is not what's on our minds.

SUNDAY

6:30 a.m.: Walking into town very early for croissants. Our love is relatively new, even though we are old. We complete each other with such ease. If someone had said at the beginning, "You'll only have three years of the most perfect love," I would not have walked away, even now.

7:43 a.m.: Awake, mixing Alan's Exjade, a drug that stabilizes the iron overload from his now over 150 blood transfusions. It has to be mixed with warm apple juice and then stirred until it dissolves and taken immediately. We call it his morning elixir.

8:00 a.m.: Now the compression stockings go on—no need for me to go to the gym or lift weights! I help him to a sitting position, where he gets momentarily dizzy from the heart medications. He nestles his head between my breasts, and I scratch his back. Good morning greetings.

8:15 a.m.: This morning was a good morning. We're changing Alan's routine a bit to see if it helps with the edema in his legs. Alan's getting dressed. A white shirt today—he looks dashing. He makes himself breakfast. This morning a yogurt shake with protein powder and a croissant. And we read the *Times* together. I start with the wedding announcements, and read him any good ones aloud. This morning there were two.

9:30 a.m.: Then more meds. Heart pills and lasix for the edema. Every time he is in the hospital, edema happens and it reduces his mobility and quality of life—which is what we focus on, knowing there is nothing curative for his condition.

10:00 a.m.: I put the oxygen canister in the car and we hook it up. And off he drives in our little car with the painted roof to Mayo to get his IV. I am immensely attracted to him even when he's hooked up to IVs and has his dentures out.

10:30 a.m.: Alan does feel badly that we aren't able to be intimate, so private "orgasm sessions" seem to make sense. I masturbate every week or so, when he's not around. I turn to my neon green vibrator from Babeland. It only takes a minute or so—I've always been highly orgasmic—and it does relax me. I don't often fantasize, and when I do, it's not about Alan. It's about the professor I dated before him, who was very well-endowed. I've come to realize that sex and love can easily be decoupled. Which, I think, men know instinctively.

12:00 p.m.: My daughter called. I married her father thirty years ago when I wanted to be respectable, and I wanted another kid. On the surface our marriage looked okay, in the two-children, blazer-and-khaki traditions of Virginia. He was a serious alcoholic and womanizer. And I never knew about the latter until the end. (Him: "It never threatened the marriage; it was like going for a run in the morning." Speechless.)

1:00 p.m.: Alan just brought me home a kumquat, "a small burst of excitement," alluding to the "bursts" that no longer happen physically between us. We do miss that.

3:43 p.m.: Alan is napping. The guest chef is in the kitchen cooking gumbo for our supper guests. In the past we would have done the shopping together and made an adventure out of it. I miss the grocery store adventures and discussions about what to get. So now I'm the shopper and errand runner and working full time and managing his health care. It's almost like being a single mother—which I was for years, so it's an easy gig—except that I don't have as much energy. He still cooks though, so I am not starving.

7:00 p.m.: Enjoying dinner with friends. It is clear that he and I are made of the same stuff, despite our apparent surface differences. He sailed a boat in the Caribbean for three decades. We love to nest (a boat, remember, is a floating nest). He's the cook and I'm the cleaner-upper. I saw this on a restroom stall door: *I don't know what souls are made of, but ours are the same.*

11:04 p.m.: Great dinner party. A treat. I am reminded over and over again of his humor and wit. I will miss him terribly.

MONDAY

7:01 a.m.: Early early. Tea about to boil. Going for a walk. Alan is sleeping. He is more fatigued and still battling edema, and I hope nothing else. He may need a transfusion and blood work today. A reminder of his frailty.

7:19 a.m.: I've been married three times. The first was at 19. If marrying for lust, he was the guy: a blue-eyed square jawed punter on an Ivy League football team. My mother said that when you loved someone, fireworks happened and you got married and lived happily ever after. (Had I paid attention to my parent's marriage, I would've known she was glossing.) We had plenty of sex which I was enthusiastic about, and never an orgasm. Didn't know what I was missing. I left him right after the baby. He was having an affair, unemployed, and playing a lot of golf. I had an epiphany: I could take care of myself and the baby, but I wasn't babysitting a grownup.

9:00 a.m.: Alan is quite self-sufficient. The less obvious and more taxing stuff: monitoring ten different medications twice a day. Taking his temperature and blood pressure in the morning. Monitoring the liquid oxygen level in the tank. Checking his oxygen saturation levels with an oximeter frequently throughout the day. Getting his oxygen set up for the car. Maintaining a spreadsheet with all medications, procedures, transfusions, hospitalizations. And learning about the interactions now that more of his systems are failing. Example: letting the urology doctor know that he can't rely on the white blood count because the cancer has elevated it. But living with a man who has little time left makes the small stuff much smaller.

12:07 p.m.: Doing a dry run with the sixtyish woman who will come to help Alan for the next two days, as I am off to see my dying mother. I will be gone for two days and am nervous. She will help Alan in the morning and at night, though he still needs to drive himself to Mayo. It's time for the medic alert button.

10:09 p.m.: I make sure pads are in our bed in case of night sweats.

10:23 p.m.: Off to bed. We do the compression stocking removal, which is fairly orgasmic. Think the scene from *When Harry Met Sally*. And since he has two legs, multiple orgasms. We have fun.

10:40 p.m.: Often at night I massage his feet before we go to bed. He is the love of my life.

11:00 p.m.: During the night, we cuddle mostly with our feet and legs—his spleen is swollen and uncomfortable to touch, and he has a catheter line in one arm, so I'm always conscious of being careful even in my sleep. Sometimes he rests his hand on my head and massages my scalp.

11:08 p.m.: I do not see myself entering into another serious relationship, ever. I had been looking for him all my life—and I found him. So when he's done, I'm done. I imagine I will live a long time, but my energies will go elsewhere. We have chosen our grave site and ordered our marker. It's made of glass. Our last nest.

PART THREE

poly

7

cheating

ON PAPER, I'M MONOGAMOUS, IN PRACTICE. . .

During my wonderful marriage, I did have a number of casual sexual encounters, mostly overseas. Edie and I never talked about it, but she was an extremely intelligent woman, and I'm pretty sure she knew.

—The Newly Widowed Player

She didn't know! She totally didn't know!

—Anonymous reader

There are only two topics that draw more divisive responses than politics: chiropractics and cheating. At any dinner party, bring either topic up and you are doomed, because the table is ringed with people who have been touched by either and claim harm.

Of course, given my job, infidelity is the first topic that people bring up: "Do you see cheating a lot in the diaries?" "What causes infidelity?" "Any good anecdotes?" Which is how I know that announcing, "So, is anyone in here currently cheating?" is a great way to silence a room.

The answer? Likely no. Cheating is much less common than you'd think. Surveys consistently find that only 4% of married people cheat per year. There's some indication that younger generations cheat a bit more, but even then, in a lifetime, 18% of men and 15% of women say they have had intercourse outside their marriage; some estimates are as high as a quarter, but still, that's in a *lifetime*. The gender difference is due to logistics—it's trickier for a busy mom to cheat than a traveling dad.[1]

The diaries are a trove of perspective on cheating, beginning with how it gets detected in the first place. Male diarists frequently suspect that they are being cheated on, citing "just a sense" that their partner is doing them wrong . . . and they are almost always incorrect. As one 35-year-old diarist wrote, "I think that she has too many male friends that she communicates with on a daily basis." This may well be true, but he's not pointing out any specific evidence of cheating. When female diarists suspect cheating, they are almost always correct, and it is because they are pinpointing specific evidence or a change in behavior: The Artist Mom points out that her husband always asks about his mistress first when making social plans, and "whenever they're together, she'll find any excuse to touch him."

And when caught, it is almost always, without fail, by cell phone. Yes, people: If you are behaving suspiciously, your partner is going to look on your cell phone.

So what *is* cheating? Diaries are internal monologues, and the line between what diarists *consider* doing versus actually *do* is very thin, and in many cases, a matter of chance. Take The Editor Considering Leaving Her Husband. She has been faithful for her entire marriage, and makes it quite clear that given the opportunity to cheat with her beloved, she would. Or The Octogenarian with Many Many Secrets who is pious, even fidelitious. He has been with his wife for six decades, and a perfect husband for the last twenty. But he still spends many daily hours reliving past sexual memories of his former, longtime mistress. Are they cheating?

The line is further confused because of the outside judgment involved in deeming someone a cheater. A sex act by itself is largely meaningless: we, as a culture, only care *who* is doing it. The exact same behaviors you're about to read between a married couple wouldn't raise an eyebrow. Yet the reaction that many readers have to the tawdry disclosures of The Newly Widowed Player isn't to *what* he's doing (vanilla sex), but to *whom* he is doing it with (married women) and considering doing it with (the wives of friends).

After reading the inner monologues of numerous cheaters, I no longer think of cheating in terms of who did what, and I've stopped parsing the line between sexual and emotional cheating. Many diarists think these thoughts, so I would instead like to reframe the discussion to look at why diarists are creating these boundaries in their lives in the first place, particularly the ones that cause them to be dishonest with their partners.

Lovers: Not the Cheating Kind

There is a pattern to cheating, which helps make sense of things. Lovers rarely, if ever, cheat. I've never seen it. And it's not because these diarists don't ever stray. Far from it—Lovers are highly sexual diarists, who do sometimes have sex outside the primary relationship without permission from their partner. But Lover relationships are built on a foundation of immediate honesty, and these diarists tend to disclose their slip ups to their partner fairly quickly—at which point it's no longer cheating. Sure, there are deep relationship consequences: sometimes they breakup, sometimes endless therapy ensues, sometimes the relationship opens up. Often though, these diarists disclose their attractions to their partner long before cheating occurs.

The complete lack of cheating among Lovers helps pinpoint what is so damaging about cheating in the first place. Contrary to popular opinion, sleeping with someone else (or considering sleeping with, or forging an emotional connection with) is not the problem. The problem is the violation of the primary relationship agreement. It's not about the sex; it's about the lying about the sex. The Successful Consultant in the previous chapter recalls her ex-husband saying that sleeping with his mistress was "just like going for a run." It probably was. The runs were not what imploded his relationship; the rampant concealing of the truth was. Similarly, The Jekyll-and-Hyde Grad Student belongs in this chapter not because of his extracurricular activities, but because he hasn't *told* his girlfriend about his extracurricular activities. Cheating is a communication failure. You'll see these diarists cavalierly justify their dishonesty, like The Newly Widowed Player, who tells himself that his wife knew. Keep in mind that "cheating" means to act dishonestly or unfairly in order to achieve an advantage; to deceive or trick.

Cheating is the domain of Partners and Aspirers, and appears in the diaries in two very different forms, which I'll describe below. To distinguish, I like to ask each cheating diarist a question: Do you feel that you're partnered with the right person? No, I'm Not Partnered with the Right Person

Diarists like The Octogenarian could trademark the line, "I'm not the kind of person who cheats." They often write pages saying that they simply had no idea that they could feel this way, and are genuinely dumbfounded to find that connections of passion exist at all. These surprise attractions often result in long-term, emotionally involved affairs. Many diarists in the book are in this scenario: The Finance Dad in Chapter 3 left his Partner marriage for his Aspirer mistress; The Minister in Chapter 6 would, in a heartbeat, begin a spiritually laced Lover affair if the right woman appeared. The core issue is that the diarist wants a whole different *type* of relationship.

Partners are less likely to stray in the first place—sex is not a high priority—and when they do, it is often because they have unexpectedly found a highly charged physical/spiritual/intellectual Lover connection. They are absolutely stunned at the turn of events. We begin now in Toronto with a seasoned infidel who experienced just that.

The Octogenarian with Many, Many Secrets

87, Toronto, Canada, Partner

FRIDAY

8:00 a.m.: Watch Mass. It's an excellent Roman Catholic Mass. I couldn't do without it. My wife still goes every day.

9:00 a.m.: Wife returns from mass. She is 85, and is in better health than I am now. So we have a Filipino girl help us here now, and she has prepared us breakfast.

10:00 a.m.: My wife is really very kind to me. She just gave me a sponge bath, because I came out of the hospital yesterday with the possibility of leaving this Earth. It was silent. Well, "The water is fine" and "Thank you" and that kind of thing. Our sixty years of marriage seems incredible.

10:30 a.m.: I watch Regis and Kelly until I have enough strength again. Then I go to the computer and look at what has come in. I keep in touch with people all over the world.

4:00 p.m.: Oprah.

9:00 p.m.: Bedtime. We have two twin beds. I go to bed when I want to, and she likes to go to bed later.

9:32 p.m.: I am looking forward to Monday morning: the nurse comes by to give me a shower and wash my total body and puts grease on my private parts!

SATURDAY

9:00 a.m.: The girl came to give me a shower. I have very little power. Now we are off to a funeral.

3:35 p.m.: I feel unbelievable. Today I saw Sophie. She was so busy organizing everything related to the funeral. Her husband is famous, and it was her mother-in-law's funeral. But she was kind to my wife. I hadn't seen her in at least a year. So seeing her again really meant a lot to me. It was unbelievable.

3:38 p.m.: I remember when we had our first encounter. I had met her at a party at my place in the country, and then drove six hours to see her. We had tea and went for a nice walk in the sunshine and after dinner we went to bed. It seemed no problem that I joined her. She was expecting with her first child. What an experience, that lovely soft body next to me. Well developed breasts in my hands, her head on my shoulder, something that I had never experienced before. My tongue surrounded her nipples and sucked them with pleasure which she liked so much.

6:40 p.m.: It is interesting that after these many years I can get aroused but then cannot fulfill my feelings with anyone. I can remember how nice it was when I felt her soft skin and soft breasts and sucked her nipples, which she loved.

7:00 p.m.: We loved to be in each other's arms. Love based on friendship, which was something very new to me. Seeing her again reminded me of that fantastic meaningful relationship.

SUNDAY

9:30 a.m.: My wife has brought me communion. She is kind and does good things, but can say unbelievably hard things. We never fell in love. I didn't, anyway. Did she? Seems so. She says she still loves me. And then I met Sophie. And that's the reason why I have this feeling.

10:00 a.m.: The girl is helping me with my injections. And then I'm on the computer, working very heavily on family trees, and my memoirs.

12:15 p.m.: I really love Sophie. I really love her. She's in her fifties now.

12:18 p.m.: That way of spontaneous sex—no forcing each other to do things neither wanted to do. It was an unbelievable way of sharing. It was spontaneous. We saw each other three or four times a week, sometimes a couple times a day. At the end of ten years, it was like married life together. I've never written about all this kind of stuff. It's good to get rid of it.

1:00 p.m.: My wife made lunch. Often, my wife's touching would bother me. And I am a hugger! The more the better, and lots of kisses.

4:00 p.m.: Just spoke on the phone for an hour with a friend of forty years. In my life there are many female friends who give me a lot of pleasure, not in a sexual sense, but we are able to discuss the inners in our life without being embarrassed about it. I talk to people about Sophie.

4:01 p.m.: I remember we had once gone to a convention in a hotel and stayed there over night, and in the morning my wife left and Sophie came to visit me. It didn't take very long and we were involved in a stormy sex scene. I entered her and she screamed of enjoyment. I had never experienced such an event.

4:03 p.m.: At one time I felt masturbation was a way of doing it, but not now. Don't forget that I am deeply religious.

4:10 p.m.: My wife and I don't talk about sex. Indeed, a real sex event would be pleasant. A steaming event where we suck each other and then relax for a while and then try it again, starting from the toes up!

6:00 p.m.: Usually my wife makes dinner, but now we have this Filipino girl, and my wife is teaching her.

9:38 p.m.: Went back to bed and asked my wife if she would join me. She said NO.

MONDAY

9:00 a.m.: The girl came in to do my shower. And just so you know, no, I don't want her to do anything. I'm very close to her.

10:00 a.m.: Wife returns. I think she finds that she gets more out of church than before.

12:00 p.m.: I feel better today. We do errands. My wife can drive a long distance in the car, and we won't say a word together. Not a word. Pleasant silence. Sometimes she says something sarcastic, but I don't react to it. That aggravates her more.

4:00 p.m.: Thinking again. That's what I do now. I had Sophie for ten years. The family was upset, though some understood. My daughters, they are in their fifties. They do not know the full extent. And, well, my wife, she went to Sophie's place and gave her hell. Whatever a woman does to another woman. I don't know if her husband knew. Her husband was a good friend of mine, and still is. He probably knew something was going on. My friend upstairs [God] said, "You can get an annulment, except I don't agree with that."

9:00 p.m.: I am always happy to go to sleep at night and have my relationship with my Maker.

TUESDAY

9:31 a.m.: My wife has made me breakfast, in silence. It has been difficult; we can't share things very easily. We were separated for two years because of all of this. I had all the divorce papers prepared. Sophie and I ended because we didn't want to hurt two families. And it became difficult for Sophie because people would be in the house looking after the family. Relatives. If you say you're going to end it, you have to end it, because otherwise it only aggravates the feelings.

10:43 a.m.: Resting on my bed. It is interesting that over the years I always have tried to have our bedroom facing east. That morning sunshine makes one feel better. I have two little ones in heaven there. One was born with an open head. So she is our angel in heaven.

10:45 a.m.: Sophie had a third child. I was very keen on that child, very very keen. That child is very much in my mind every day. We never had protected sex. So it has been. I joined Big Brothers Big Sisters, and got a boy the same age. And that boy and Sophie's boy became very good friends. Now he is 31. But one day Sophie was trying to cross the highway, and a motorcycle came over the bridge, and hit that car. So my little boy was instantly dead. He was the only one who died. I was absolutely caput. So he's an angel out the window now.

2:00 p.m.: Day out for lunch with Jeanine, a girl I met at the bank when I needed to open a bank account. I've always had close friends. I have lunch and talk about everything under the sun. My wife sometimes feels that's funny. But none could ever compare with Sophie. No way.

2:15 p.m.: I won't do anything with finances, even buy a car, unless I talk to Jeanine. I need the playback, the feedback. It's painful if you can't have that from the person you're married to. Particularly if there's some kind of hurtful comment back.

7:34 p.m.: Technology has had a positive influence on my life. I still keep in touch with my real estate clients and often advise them with their investments. Gadgets keep me occupied.

WEDNESDAY

9:00 a.m.: No strength today. In 2009, we had a renewal of our vows. I felt I had to do that, and my friend above told me to. I do not know why I started my marriage. I guess I needed someone to be with. I made up my mind that we will make it work, no matter the obstacles and difficulties. It's always easier to give up, and think that a different person would make it better and simpler. My friend upstairs is my greatest help in these situations.

9:16 a.m.: Presently I am getting replies from distant family members about our family tree. In 1949 I got married, but to my surprise never fell in love. We had a huge wedding. When I left after the dinner, I felt sorry I was missing all these people. As a matter of fact, I cried. My father gave us a car and we went to a hotel. They gave us champagne. And then my first experience was horrible. Horrible. It was a total bloodbath. Which I now know is normal, but did not know that would be the case. But now I feel happy because I have been able to tackle the difficulties in our relationship. One has to overcome the negatives that seem to exist.

2:00 p.m.: Today had a nice lunch with a male friend I used to work with at the firm. He has been married three times, and this time it is an unbelievable relationship. It's nice to see when people are happy.

9:52 p.m.: It might be surprising to you that after I have given you the insight of my thoughts that my main strength comes from my special friend upstairs, and many of my friends who have joined Him. After my heart attacks, doctors expected me to pass away, but still I am smiling and still here. ***

Yes, I'm Partnered with the Right Person: I'm Just Having Sex on the Side

Cheating diarists like The Jekyll-and-Hide Dirty Grad Student and The Newly Widowed Player are happy at home. Their Partner or Aspirer relationship fulfills many needs, adrenaline-filled sex notwith-standing—a fact which the diarists use to justify their no-strings-attached dalliances. Emotional attachment with a mistress is never the aim; if emotional attachment does arise, the diarist often states, from the beginning, that he or she is not going to leave their partner.

Aspirer diarists like The Newly Widowed Player are opportunists, and much more likely to cheat when assured that their family life is not at risk. Many use sex workers, as do two of the diarists in this chapter. They are far from alone—the entire prostitution industry is substantially supported by infidelity. The most reliable numbers indicate that twenty percent of men over forty say they've paid for sex.[2]

Note that *none* of the diarists in this chapter are cheating in response to some lack in their primary partner; in fact, every diarist adores their partner. The Newly Widowed Player absolutely loved his wife. When reading his diary, it hits you how not-a-big-deal cheating is for him, because in his mind it is a purely sexual encounter, and not a threat to his primary relationship. (His spouse, of course, would feel otherwise.) It's just one small part of his life.

The Newly Widowed Player Who Kept a Huge Secret from His Wife of 50 Years

80, Sarasota, Florida

FRIDAY

8:01 a.m.: Busy day ahead. I wonder if Frances will call again. Tough to get her out of mind after last week. But what about Jack?

10:30 a.m.: Lunch with the guys. If I don't hear from Frances, I'll give her a call before her husband Jack gets home. Beginning to think that maybe it was not a good idea to visit them.

3:53 p.m.: Frances just called. Sounded as confused as I am. Our first sex was 56 years ago, when I was single and she was married. She says she misses me making her feel desirable. Almost fell off the chair when she suggested that a *ménage-à-trois* might be good. Exciting— but with Jack? Now I'm sitting here with an erection.

4:00 p.m.: Maybe Frances thinks that now that my wife has died, we should start again. Our mutual oral sex last week was really great. I gotta say, for a couple of codgers, we do pretty well. Don't know where this is going.

7:25 p.m.: Nothing on the schedule for tonight. I think I'll read for a while, watch the news and go to bed. Evenings are tough. I miss Edie so much and am so lonely. I miss talking with her and holding her while watching what she likes on TV. She really understands me. We both assumed that I was going to go first. This isn't the way it should be.

SATURDAY

6:00 a.m.: Early mornings are difficult, too. Edie died six months and two days ago. The first couple of months were extremely difficult. I occasionally get emotional when anything comes up that's reminiscent of times we've had together—last week it was driving through mountains. She was very fond of mountainous areas. We were married for 55 years, and we started out with literally nothing, and managed to gather wonderful friends, two children, and very many wonderful memories.

8:13 a.m.: Tough getting moving today—and not a hell of a lot to get moving for. Would be pretty great to share these last years, to get below the surface with someone.

10:32 a.m.: Putzing around day. Maybe I'll make a pot of soup, and later I'll give Marty and Ruth a call to see if anything interesting is going on.

12:00 p.m.: Bumped into Miri at the dry cleaners. She's looking good. Is it usual to get aroused by married women? It might be because I'm really horny since last week's visit to Frances.

7:08 p.m.: Mentioned my dinner plans to Skip, down the hall. He kidded me about women. Suggested I check out Craigslist to find one. Told him I wasn't interested in an STD.

9:43 p.m.: Just got back—good dinner. Noah is not as sharp as my other friends, but still a good conversation. Edie enjoyed them, too—well, maybe "tolerated" them. God, she was the love of my life.

SUNDAY

7:00 a.m.: I feel shitty. Edie was in the nursing facility with Alzheimer's for two years, and I went over every morning, and three times a day, for a total of six hours a day. Every day I realize just how much she means to me, even now. From our first date, Edie and I had the greatest relationship any couple could hope to have. No matter whether we were together or apart, doing something serious or silly, by ourselves or with others, there was always a connection. We just really loved each other, and were always trying to do something to please the other. Even if I had it to do all over again, I wouldn't change a thing.

8:52 a.m.: Meeting Hans and Esther for our usual brunch buffet. Might be a good time to hint around that I'd be open to meeting some single ladies. Other than this situation with Frances, I haven't dated at all.

8:55 a.m.: Edie and I both really enjoyed intimacy, all sorts of sexual items. Of course I'm speaking for her, but I think she did. Probably two to three times a week. I spent most of my career traveling, and if

I was gone for a couple of days, we'd make up for it. When we retired, there was a slackening to maybe once a week. I never realized how important physical contact is to me.

12:00 p.m.: Here's an idea: Maybe I'll go down to the beach and check out the young ladies. The fresh air will be good and some nice bodies in bikinis will give me something to think about later.

4:53 p.m.: The beach was good. I enjoyed looking at the 20-something hard bodies. Too bad they didn't come out with thongs when I was much younger.

6:00 p.m.: Enjoyed the shower when I got home. That body wash lubricated the right place! A little self-indulgence is good.

7:58 p.m.: I don't have any plans for this evening. I think I'll have a little snack and go back to the Nora Roberts book that Frances gave me last week. She said she was sure I'd enjoy it.

8:59 p.m.: Now I know why! Some pretty steamy scenes. It is a good thing we are 1,500 miles apart. That's temptation with a capital T! A long long time ago, before I was married, she and I had a rather torrid affair. Whenever the opportunity presented itself, we found a way to be together. And then, after I was married, I very carefully avoided the situation for a good ten years or so.

9:00 p.m.: I honestly don't remember the details, but somewhere along the line we hooked up again. We lived in different states, and infrequently, there would be a chance to get together. From a purely sexual viewpoint, she's one of the most exciting ladies I've ever been with. Her enjoyment of whatever happens to be happening really turns me on. We had oral sex this time. There was a great deal of concern on her part, and mine as well, that Jack would be home soon.

10:00 p.m.: Talked to our "kids" (mid-50s) and grandkids. They sound pretty good.

MONDAY

9:30 a.m.: Bumped into the cleaning girl in the hall a few minutes ago, and another was at the elevator waiting for her. As we rode down the elevator, my mind leaped immediately to a threesome. I think it would be really interesting to spend several hours with two women, both about 5'3", about 110 lbs., dark hair, blue eyes, average to slightly small breasts.

Various positions, oral sex, and whatever else comes to mind. Perhaps if one of the two were dominant it might be even more interesting.

9:31 a.m.: These two in the elevator don't meet all the criteria I specified, but they are young (about 30), so let's not get too fussy!

12:00 p.m.: Looking forward to tomorrow. Good odds that Frances will call. This is obviously going nowhere, unless there's an opportunity for some great sex, which is questionable. Maybe I'll settle for phone sex. Knowing her, she'll be up for it.

4:40 p.m.: Spent the afternoon rebalancing my portfolio, and now am poolside. Several contemporaries there, as well as younger visitors—three female. I do like the bikinis. Good thing I put my sunglasses on after I got out of the water.

Wouldn't mind a quickie.

4:42 p.m.: Traveling as I did, the opportunities for such things certainly were there. Some of my business associates made sure they were. And it was—I'll call it "adventuresome." During my wonderful marriage, I did have a number of casual sexual encounters, mostly overseas in Europe and the Far East. Edie and I never talked about it, but she was an extremely intelligent woman, and I'm pretty sure she knew. Inasmuch as they were sexual gratification only, it didn't make much of a difference one way or another. No emotional content, just good sex. I just enjoyed it.

5:05 p.m.: Well, there was one female lawyer. I guess this was in the early 1990s that I did become quite attached to. But she understood the situation as well as I did.

6:16 p.m.: I wonder if a connection with a woman might be a good idea. The road ahead isn't long. I remember what Steve said when he observed the local ladies fussing over me—"Watch out for the casserole women!"

TUESDAY

9:58 a.m.: Met five former neighbors for breakfast. Caught up on all the news: who has moved, who has died. We stay away from relationships.

1:08 p.m.: The cleaning girl will clean my place tomorrow. I just told her that if she comes early enough, she might catch me in the shower. Her response: "Don't worry. I'll be on time."

3:12 p.m.: Quiet evening at home ahead. Set up a lunch date with Rob and Miri. I don't think Miri will be joining us. Maybe I can get a hug with her when I pick him up. Ah, you horny old man!

7:30 p.m.: Now I'm feeling the start of an erection and I really think I'm going to masturbate. I do it maybe three times a week. I have checked out a couple of porn sites and found them rather unrealistic.

9:00 p.m.: Texting my kids. Cell phones really do help us stay in touch.

WEDNESDAY

2:55 p.m.: Frances called. Glad she did. As expected, the conversation turned to sex early on, and as usual I ended up being totally aroused—which I relieved before beginning this entry.

2:57 p.m.: I really feel for her. I think she is not satisfied in a bunch of ways, but there isn't much I (we) can do about it. They sleep in separate bedrooms. Easy to understand our current attraction. I always try to be sure that a woman gets as much pleasure from an encounter as I do. Jack may not provide as much as she wants (needs). I don't want to be disloyal to Jack, though. I've known him sixty years or so. Good thing we are geographically distant.

7:03 p.m.: Rob and Miri just called. They need an extra hand for the bridge gathering at their place tonight. He does have some good Scotch. Sex is like bridge: if you don't have a partner, you should have good hands.

10:06 p.m.: Just got back—I didn't screw up too badly. Pleasant buzz, should sleep well tonight. Miri is looking great, and I wonder if she senses that I'd love to have her. Enough of that.

How Relationships Weather Cheating: Aspirers

The diaries present a distinct pattern in which relationships endure cheating. Broadly speaking, Aspirer relationships tend to survive cheating, for the simple reason that they are allies—their connections are often multidimensional, and strong in other ways. The specter of nonordained sex is certainly not pleasant, but when it arises between two people who are achieving their financial, career, and family goals, the relationship can often be preserved. You have seen this numerous times in the media between political couples—yes, the cheating is devastating, but the other priorities of the relationship still stand, and when the partners are honest with themselves, in the big picture of careers and finances and children and family and love, sex-on-the-side is just a blip. They are still allies with numerous shared interests.

We begin with The Artist Mom, whose Aspirer marriage tolerates cheating; the relationship survives because it's still serving its many purposes.

The Artist Mom Whose Husband Is Also Stepping Out

28, Denver, Colorado
THURSDAY

9:29 a.m.: I've called in sick to that joke they call "my job."

11:30 a.m.: Wish my husband could come home for a quickie.

11:35 a.m.: You know, marriage vows are too vague. "In sickness and in health, for richer and for poorer." What is that really covering? Nothing. How about: "In fatness and stink, in youth and beauty, old age and wrinkles, I will overlook your choices in lovers as you shall overlook mine. I promise to be the one you can fall back on, for I alone truly love who you are, not just how you fuck."

4:00 p.m.: On Facebook. Facebook has dredged up my history. I could do without it. You leave some towns for good reason, y'know?

7:24 p.m.: I've given up hope for any sex this week. My daughter's a burgeoning preteen, and I'm beginning to see why they say infants and teenagers are hard-on killers.

7:52 p.m.: We both love our child so much—there are so many beautiful moments when I realize that she is stunning and beautiful and that my position in life is to make her life less complicated than mine—but my husband and I do not have enough alone time. If she's having a rough day, she robs us of simply being kind to each other.

10:00 p.m.: The kid. Sucked it all out of us. We literally just sat on the couch staring at the TV. And that was okay.

FRIDAY

7:41 a.m.: Yech! Dreamed of being pregnant. I have an IUD for a reason.

9:43 a.m.: IMing one of the men I slept with behind my husband's back. We've been married 2.5 years, and I made it to 2.25 without cheating. Boredom and monogamy hold hands in my relationship—he wasn't giving me any, so I went and got it myself. But I'm much too in love with him to do anything too drastic. He is my best friend. My best friend with whom I haven't had sex for almost two weeks.

2:05 p.m.: This just in, an IM from a coworker, "I should be in bed . . . with you." Really? This is year four of workplace harassment. The one time I dressed in office-type suit attire, the creepy old guy down the hall leaned into my ear at the copy machine and whispered, "You look so hot today," before touching my ass and returning to his office. Now I wear jeans and ugly sweaters.

4:35 p.m.: Picked up a very upset kid from school. At this point I know to just let her be, so I jump in the shower to unwind. I start to masturbate and relax. Fantasize about a former black lover. I have a thing for black men. They kiss like women, all soft and deep and they aren't afraid to toss you around. I love watching my skin against caramel, or chocolate.

4:40 p.m.: Daughter bursts into the bathroom, needing attention. Kids will suck the sexual energy out of you.

4:45 p.m.: Deal with her, and send her out. In a desperate attempt to feel like a sexual creature, I put on my favorite perfume and masturbate in front of the mirror. I like to watch. I talk dirty to myself under my own breath. It works. Now off to make dinner.

8:27 p.m.: So much for getting lucky tonight. He used to pick up hookers; I used to take two or three lovers a week. I've suggested an open marriage before, and he was only okay with me having girl-friends—the idea of another man's penis in me makes him more upset then the idea of my eating pussy.

SATURDAY

8:07 a.m.: I love morning sex. But I haven't had it in almost four years. I'd have to stay in bed till noon—my husband's a sleeper. I miss it, when your body is awake well before your brain has a chance to catch up. All your nerves are present for those sessions . . . Sigh.

8:08 a.m.: He used to make breakfast, too. And do other positions—he has a habit of being very vanilla, four positions and that's that. But I suppose those are things you do for a girlfriend, not a wife.

8:10 a.m.: It's not, by the way, that we don't talk about this stuff. I've just learned that confrontation about our sex life doesn't work. It's a matter of sneakily persuading him to give me more spankings.

9:00 a.m.: I still have trouble believing that my husband was single an entire year and a half before he met me. We were having lion sex on our first night together: predatory, rough, easy, perfect. There was a pause in the action after four hours, and I looked him straight in the eyes and said, "We are never allowed to be alone in Vegas together." We'd wind up married. Which is what happened.

1:32 p.m.: Got a massage to escape the oncoming teenager-ness of my kiddo. I'm beginning to think that our lack of sex life is not entirely our fault.

2:15 p.m.: March Madness is on. Again. Husband just went to the liquor store. So much for his sticking to the gym and good food routine. When I first laid eyes on him, he was rippling with muscles from being a construction guy. He's sexy when he's not sporting a gut.

2:16 p.m.: I'm keyed up and ready to go, but the only privacy I can get for a "help yourself" session is the bathroom, and frankly, it needs to be cleaned.

3:28 p.m.: Working most of my sexual frustration into this massive piece of artwork I've been trying to finish. Had a drink, and am now looking forward to dinner at my parents' house. For some reason, being around my parents makes me want my husband even more. Perhaps I can keep him interested enough to play when we get home.

8:35 p.m.: My parents' house had the expected aphrodisiac effect. We spent the evening joking with my grandmother (dirty-minded, hilarious woman). He gets really affectionate, touching my back and rubbing my shoulders a lot. He buries his face in my neck and shares secret things when no one's listening.

10:00 p.m.: Back home, he cracks another beer, has a cigar, and is watching some nature show with the kid. He certainly has his own schedule when it comes to sexual advances.

SUNDAY

7:55 a.m.: Googling "Pregnancy Signs and IUD." It's kinda got me freaked out a little. I'm off. Most people dig babies. Babies make me want to leave the room. I don't like them. Don't get me wrong, I love every cell of my daughter. But I have no interest in putting my body or my mind through that bullshit again.

11:56 a.m.: I told my husband, and his response was, "Stick to the plan, right?" If I did wind up pregnant, we would terminate. Amazing how much I can love sex, but hate the natural result.

1:07 p.m.: It doesn't bother me so much that my husband has another lover. His time with her has injected some vitality into his bedroom style. I think we're both kidding ourselves to believe that a completely monogamous relationship will work.

1:09 p.m.: People put too much emphasis on having an emotional connection with your lover. Having sex can be just sex, and you can still go home to the one you love.

1:15 p.m.: What bothers me is his denial. I'd be alright if he said, "Yeah, I'm sleeping with her." Or even admit he's attracted to her. But he doesn't.

1:18 p.m.: And God, when I am around her, she talks about my daughter. A lot. Gives away just how much time she's been around my family that he doesn't tell me about. Yes, that part makes me murderous.

1:20 p.m.: My solution is to just not think too much about it . . . and occasionally take a lover myself.

5:39 p.m.: Bless my husband. He has managed to take my twisted, stressed-out state and turn it around. He may be a guy's guy, but when it counts, he's right on target: he did the dishes, gave me a smoke and a couple of drinks, massaged my shoulders and assured me that everything will be fine, and tossed a ball around with our daughter in the park.

8:05 p.m.: At a bar, waiting for my husband, who had to stick his head into work. I was always the dangerous one at the bar. Not because

I am the prettiest girl in the room, but rather because I'm the sexiest and most self assured.

8:15 p.m.: Margaritas and a mariachi band at our table singing "Por Amor." We've been so touchy-feely with each other all day. I keep picturing myself mounting him right there in the restaurant, with the mariachi band playing on.

MONDAY

7:34 a.m.: Whew! Not pregnant. Just really stressed out. Thank goodness. I wish having my tubes tied wasn't so expensive. I would've done it years ago.

9:09 a.m.: Having dodged that bullet, my sex drive has come roaring back. And here I am at the office.

10:40 a.m.: I've discovered a song that makes you want to drag your partner into the nearest coat closet and give him a blowjob. Yes, I am the kind of woman who likes giving head. Too many women see that as a chore, when in reality, it's a gift they can't get without you. If you look at it like "I am a freakin' porn star" and thoroughly like doing it, he'll thank you. Use a little (*a little*) honey and just go to town.

10:42 a.m.: Sending dirty little texts to my husband. I'm supposed to be working, but instead, I'm thinking about his perfect penis. It's beautiful. I would like to shake the hand of whatever doctor circumcised him.

11:20 a.m.: I am really wound up. IMing with my former fuck buddy is not keeping me grounded. He wants to meet over drinks. That way, we're in public and won't do anything. He's trying to be a good boy with his new girl, and I applaud his efforts.

12:38 p.m.: Telling my coworker to shut up about doing bad things in the empty storeroom.

2:30 p.m.: Thinking randomly about my soul mate. I found my soul's other half years ago, but circumstances forced me to let go and tell him goodbye. But he was one that I will find in the next life, and I've worked a long time to accept that.

2:36 p.m.: The man I am married to now is the love of my life because he is who I am making a life with. I am willing to work through almost anything with him. He gets me. And we laugh. At everything. That is the single most outstanding thing about him. Despite all the issues, I'm still madly in love with him, and could go on about him for pages.

4:44 p.m.: My husband has abandoned the house for his buddies and a bar tonight. Can't say that I blame him. I just hope he's up for something tonight. I'm feeling restless.

7:18 p.m.: His playing at the bar wouldn't bother me so much, except I'm pretty sure he's sleeping with the wealthy girlfriend of one of his friends. I know, I've stepped out too. But she bothers me. He swears it's not like that, but whenever they're together, she'll find any excuse to touch him when she thinks I'm not paying attention. And she's the first one he asks about when making social plans.

7:20 p.m.: His choice of her makes me wonder what it says about me. Would I be more of a turn on if I made more money? I've learned not to say anything about her at all. He jumps to her defense immediately. I cannot wait to move far away from her.

7:25 p.m.: Calming myself by remembering what my mentor told me years ago: "Never cut yourself off from love, even if it comes from another woman. If it's love, embrace it. The only person you have to answer to is you." And the only person he has to answer to is him.

9:42 p.m.: He came home.

1:45 a.m.: We ended up having a lovely evening just smokin' and talkin' and laughing together. We just click. He gets me, and sees through my usual bullshit. We laid next to each other, touching and stroking, and then laughed because we were both too worn out to carry through. We fell asleep with our hands on each other's bits, and woke up still touching hours later.

The Editor Considering Walking out on Her Husband on Easter Weekend

40, Gloucester County, New Jersey

FRIDAY

7:44 a.m.: This morning I have a headache. I am tired and I am thinking about leaving my husband.

8:38 a.m.: A few months ago I started communicating with Duane, a guy I dated in high school and was engaged to for a short time in college. He's married, too. I was unhappy, and in a matter of weeks, things progressed from "How have you been?" to "I've always loved you and still do." Obviously this caused problems in my marriage.

9:36 a.m.: Today I'm home with the kids, taking a day off. Rich is at work. We've been together for 9 years and I thought we always would be. He promises to work on our issues, and has already made a lot of changes.

10:31 a.m.: Looking at all of the photos of us together. I feel terror at the thought that I will waste my life stuck in my marriage for another 14 years until the kids are grown. What if I don't have as many years left as I think I do?

1:24 p.m.: My mom just called. She is more involved than I would prefer, because Rich apparently called her asking for advice.

1:30 p.m.: I do confide in her some. Just not the part about how I've loved Duane since I was 17, and he's the love of my life. He still makes me feel like #1 in his life, and I can trust him 100%, which seems rarer the older I get. He makes me laugh, which is big for me.

3:00 p.m.: Facebooking. At first I thought it would just be a fun thing to do casually, but I reconnected with my old flame, and it's threatening to derail my marriage. It's really affecting my life. It has been four days since I emailed Duane, as I promised in marriage therapy this week, and it was unbelievably hard at first, but now I feel like I can handle it.

10:15 p.m.: Rich just made some more moves toward me in bed. I know he is anxious to have sex again, but I don't feel like we're getting along well enough yet.

2:15 a.m.: I can't sleep at night. I worry what will happen to my kids—they're both under ten. But knowing that Duane loves me and we could be happy together if things were different fills almost every moment of my waking hours with regret. I don't want to get to the end of my life and know I didn't grab happiness with both hands when the opportunity arose.

SATURDAY

7:41 a.m.: Woke up thinking about how much time in the last few years I've spent unhappy. I need to make a decision about whether or not to stay married so that I can move forward.

7:48 a.m.: We are all headed to my brother's house a few hours away for Easter. My brother is becoming a member of the Catholic Church. My parents aren't happy, but I think it's great that he's going to be a part of his kids' spiritual lives. My husband does not like my brother or hanging out at others' houses, but he is making more of an effort to be there for me, so he's coming. We'll see how it goes.

1:00 p.m.: Sitting on a hard church pew watching my brother get baptized, daydreaming about Duane. I might be remembering it as something better than it was at this point, but I think it was the best relationship I've ever had. He always put me first, and when we decided to have sex for our first times, we waited until after graduation and we loved it and did it constantly all summer. Then I left for college and he stayed behind to work. By the time I found out I was pregnant, I had broken up with him. I had an abortion without telling him and have always regretted it. Not so much the abortion, since it allowed me to get an education. But I do regret not telling him and not staying with him, because he was such a great guy.

7:49 p.m.: My brother is now Catholic.

11:00 p.m.: Hotel. Rich's snoring is so much better now that he lost 30 pounds. I really appreciate the fact that he (finally) was willing to lose weight so that we can sleep in the same bed. We slept in separate rooms for three years. I actually liked it since I could get a good night's sleep every night. Sharing a bed now is tough.

SUNDAY

6:00 a.m.: Got about five hours of sleep before the kids woke up and wanted to check out their Easter baskets. Adorable.

12:54 p.m.: At my brother's house. They did a great job with brunch and the Easter egg hunt, and they have a nice big house to hang out in—though every time we see them they are looking for a larger, newer house. They are very into appearances. I feel like my mom passed that trait along to both of us. I try to fight it but I find myself feeling like what I have is inadequate.

1:58 p.m.: Find myself thinking about Duane. Maybe he's just someone who will stay in my mind for years and pop up when I least expect it. I know deep down that we won't be together unless one of us takes our children away from our spouse and moves, which I'm not willing to do and I know he's not either.

10:15 p.m.: Just nicely turned Rich down for sex again. I need to have my emotional needs met before I can consider sex. It's frustrating that there are things we need to work on, but his focus always seems to be sex. Why does that have to be such a big part of married life? Even when it's really good, I still could do without it.

10:20 p.m.: I should say that I've explored plenty. I can say that being fairly attractive has given me more choices—I had boyfriends when my friends did not get asked out, so that might have helped my self-esteem. Though I recently found out that a guy I dated came out. Which was really surprising. Not that the sex was great—it was actually not that good at all. I went back and looked at a bunch of romantic letters he wrote me, and a few were written on pink paper. In one he mentions the movie *Beaches*.

MONDAY

7:00 a.m.: Woke up this morning after getting several hours of sleep in a row, which was fantastic since I haven't been sleeping.

8:30 a.m.: Off to work. My fulltime job is very stressful. Feeling good about today, and I'm giving one of my editors a very positive review this afternoon, which is always nice. It's great to not have to point out the things someone is doing wrong.

12:23 p.m.: Quick lunch break Facebook check. Duane is back on (he had removed his profile when I asked him to). It's comforting just to see his photo up there, even though I can't see what he's posting. I want to send him an email saying that I miss him, but won't. It's best if we don't talk, I guess.

12:56 p.m.: Lunch with my friend Kay. We talked about work and where we're going to take our vacation. I'll be lucky to take one at all, due to our finances, but I didn't say that.

1:30 p.m.: I now haven't talked to Duane in nearly a week. I can't talk about it with Kay, but after this weekend, I feel like I'm deciding to stay with my husband and work things out.

3:52 p.m.: I mentioned earlier that I feel I've turned a corner, but then this afternoon I went back and reread the last few emails that Duane sent me. Why can't I just talk to him like a friend and not get emotionally involved?

7:53 p.m.: Marriage therapy. Went pretty well. The therapist mostly focused on Rich and his relationship with his mom and how it affects us. It was nice to be off the hook, given that my correspondence with Duane has taken up quite a bit of therapy time.

9:00 p.m.: I wouldn't have said this a few weeks ago, but I think this weekend I turned a corner, and have decided to try to do everything I can to make my marriage work.

9:10 p.m.: Though if Duane emailed me tomorrow and said he was flying in from Colorado, I can't say I would refuse.

How Relationships Weather Cheating: Partners

Unlike Aspirers, Partners are exquisitely vulnerable to both breakups and divorce. Partner relationships are rooted in a comfortable sense of ownership over each other's bodies, which Partner diarists verbalize often. The Lovestruck College Kid wrote, "My body is only mine and hers. Her body is only mine." The Blissfully Boring Waitress points out, "We find ourselves jealous of previous significant others." Imagine what happens when that significant other enters the present tense. Which is why cheating particularly devastates Partners—they perceive cheating to mean that their partner isn't a partner at all, but a traitor. When that ownership is suddenly destroyed, the other partner frequently runs for the hills, seeing it as the ultimate betrayal.

Next up is The Jekyll-and-Hyde Dirty Grad Student. The day that his girlfriend finds out about his Craigslist activities (which, let's say it all together: she's going to discover on his cell phone) will also be the last day of his relationship.

The Jekyll-and-Hyde Dirty Grad Student

27, Harlem, New York

TUESDAY

6:00 a.m: At university gym. There are two girls I always like seeing in the morning. One is a 6-foot blonde, and another a 5-foot brunette. I have varying tastes. Good workout!

7:00 a.m: Get back from workout and I am really horny. Get onto porn site. Search for transsexual porn. I am into guys, girls, and TS [transsexuals]. Just depends on my mood. I have only dated girls though, probably that Midwest guilt. Masturbate to a dominatrix scene I stumble across.

7:30 a.m.: I have this habit of searching Craigslist Casual Encounters while I'm looking at porn. Often times, I respond to ads when I am horny. This has led to my three transsexual encounters, and several other interesting experiences. I decide I am going to put up an ad this time, looking for a woman to have sex with me with a strap-on. I have been really into dominatrix stuff lately.

8:00 a.m: Head off to the lab, wondering if I am a little too much into sex.

4:00 p.m.: Almost end of the day, keep checking email. Nothing.

6:00 p.m.: Head to girlfriend's apartment. Immediately start up. This girl is a lot more sexual than my previous girlfriend and loves having sex all the time. I finish with her lying flat on the bed and me behind her, my favorite position with her as she has an awesome big ass. She doesn't climax. Only the second or third time this has happened. Ugh.

10:00 p.m.: Cuddle with girlfriend in bed. Why do girls like this so much?

WEDNESDAY

6:00 a.m.: Wake up with girlfriend and cuddle a little more.

6:30 a.m.: Go for a run. Thinking about what a MWM threesome would be like. I think I would enjoy that, but I have had no luck setting it up so far.

8:00 a.m.: In lab, lamenting the fact that I am not having sex.

10:00 a.m.: Masturbate in secluded bathroom. When I was with my last girlfriend, this was almost an everyday occurrence.

THURSDAY

7:45 a.m.: Wake up late, immediately head to computer. Find some solid transsexual porn and masturbate.

8:00 a.m.: Check my special email, and I have a response from a dominatrix who wants to shoot a video. Look at her web site. Respond eagerly.

8:05 a.m.: See a Craigslist ad for a girl giving sexual massages, and she has an amazing rack. Send email. This is how Craigslist works: either everything happens at once, or nothing.

9:00 a.m.: Send emails back and forth with dominatrix. She is a hot, short, petite brunette with a nice rack. The video she is making is for her website and will be for sale online. Hesitate to respond. Think what the hell, and respond anyway. We set it up for early afternoon.

11:00 a.m.: Call massage girl. She says she wants me to get a hotel room. I say no, because the "massage" is $200. She says she'll let me know.

12:00 p.m.: Massage girl, via text, agrees to come to my apartment. Weird.

1:00 p.m.: Head to meet dominatrix. This is ridiculous, and it shows how far my sexuality has come. I was really reserved sexually for the first 22 years of my life in the Midwest.

1:30 p.m.: Dominatrix calls me to tell me we may have to postpone. I already left lab to meet her at Starbucks.

1:35 p.m.: Dominatrix calls, says she will meet me at Starbucks in twenty. I call massage girl and make up some bullshit about class. She's upset, but says she will meet me later. Wow, this is going to be the most ridiculous day I have ever had.

2:00 p.m.: Meet S (dominatrix) at Starbucks. Really hot. Walk with her to her friend's apartment for the shoot.

3:00 p.m.: Set everything up, and she gets into her outfit and puts me into a pair of female panties and a dog collar. Real hot. Sign paperwork, etc.

3:15 p.m.: Shoot first scene, which is me crawling into the kitchen and then being put over her knee and spanked hard for ten minutes. I want it to stop several times because it hurts so much. Keep going anyway because there is a certain amount of pleasure in it.

3:30 p.m.: Second scene is set. In this scene, she will bend me over the kitchen table and put fingers in me. I don't get why straight guys are so afraid of ass-play, it feels amazing. Then she will use the strap-on.

4:00 p.m.: The strap-on experience is my first and it was amazing. Clean up and go home.

5:00 p.m.: Massage girl comes over. She is really busty, but also a little thick. She is young, probably 21. I like it. She changes into a sexy outfit and meets me on my bed. She gets her money upfront. She is actually massaging me, I'm surprised. Amazing rack and gives me a happy ending.

7:00 p.m.: Meet girlfriend and go to bar to meet with our two friends.

9:00 p.m.: We go back to my house and have a quickie, nothing special. I am surprised I can go again. Most ridiculous day ever.

FRIDAY

9:00 a.m.: Wake up with a hard on. Girlfriend goes down on me.

7:00 p.m.: Go out to bar with friends with girlfriend in tow. She looks amazing in a dress and heels.

10:00 p.m.: Girlfriend is drunk, which means loud. She texts me from directly next to me that she wants to suck my dick right now. I text her I want a WMW threesome with her. Doesn't seem to be into it. I figure I might as well try while she is drunk.

12:00 a.m.: Go to her house. She is now angry about something and goes right to bed. Decide to masturbate in her bathroom.

SATURDAY

9:00 a.m.: Wake up and she isn't mad. Must have been alcohol. Spoon her and we start up. I convince her to go to the shower and let me have sex with her in the ass. Yes!

11:00 a.m.: Run errands with girlfriend. She is just wearing sweats, but she still looks pretty. To be honest, she is probably out of my league. She is very pretty and smart, and from a wealthy family. I am none of those things.

5:00 p.m.: Watch a rugby game with girlfriend and my buddy. Man, I think I might actually love this chick. Can I stop my other random sexual activity and just be with her? She doesn't know about the other sexual escapades, and probably wouldn't be happy if she found out.

9:00 p.m.: Have sex with girlfriend again and finish on her skin. She likes when I finish inside, but I like finishing on her.

SUNDAY

8:00 a.m.: Get back from gym and head straight for the computer. Masturbate to a MILF, her friend, and MILF's husband. Amazing!

9:00 a.m.: Walking to school, notice one of the students I assistant-taught last semester. A 5-foot blonde. I have fantasized about her several times. It would probably be wrong to sleep with a 19-year-old.

6:00 p.m.: Pretty nonsexual day. Met girlfriend at my house for dinner.

8:30 p.m.: Ate and then had sex. Pretty good.

9:00 p.m.: Cuddle with girlfriend in my bed.

8

flourishing: the more, the merrier

One must do something to relieve the monogamy.

—Anonymous

This is my favorite chapter of the book, because it draws on the diaries that changed my life. I mention this because it irks me when I read a book, and then, a year later, read in a magazine that the author has extensive personal experience on the topic, and neglected to mention it anywhere in her 300-page book. It makes me mistrust her. Which is why I'll tell you that when I began collecting diaries back in 2007, I was a card-carrying monogamist. I was a typical late-twenty-something on the boyfriend market, not the new-lifestyle market. But over that year of five hundred diaries, I read dozens of diarists just like the ones you're about to read: diarists in stable, long-term partnerships, with one or more sexual relationships on the side. They seemed like pretty happy people.

What drew me to them was not their high-octane sex lives (though it was an attraction), but their broad webs of happy relationships, platonic and not. Each diarist seemed to be king or queen of a little world filled with loved ones, mixing platonic and romantic relationships as made sense. I emphasize this because every diarist in this book runs their bedroom the same way that they run the rest of their life, and these diarists exhibit the same creative flair in building *all* their relationships, sexual or not. Sex is just a representation of how one operates in the world.

Slowly over the years, I cherry picked from the parts of all diarists' lives that resonated, and put them into practice in my own life. And as of this writing, I've been in a long-term open relationship for three years. It's what works for me, right now.

I made this decision quietly until, while writing this book, I went home to visit my family. I stayed well within the unspoken agreement that all children and parents share that *no one* wants to know everything. Yet it was on that visit that I truly understood what it means to be closeted. My relationship is such a huge part of my life, and yet I felt misunderstood, because my family's vocabulary of "married/dating/single" didn't leave a slot for my lifestyle. (My mother: "I don't approve.") My entire life was a conceptual blank spot for her. And so my goal in this chapter is not to espouse or encourage any particular relationship style—as the previous seven chapters show, the best anyone can aim for is to meet their priorities in the way that makes sense for them—but to simply pull back the curtain on the many ways that some diarists operate their private lives from the inside.

Nonmonogamous relationships are not just widely misunderstood by mainstream culture; they're not understood *at all*. From the outside, they are assumed to be all about sex, and you wouldn't be blamed for assuming as much based on the sex-driven vocabulary that describes the subcategories: swinging (partner-swapping), polyfidelity (committed threesomes or foursomes), polyamory (simultaneous significant relationships), among many others. The sexual overtones are heightened, I think, because whenever a subgroup isn't quite understood, the mainstream oversexualizes it (i.e., hippies, AIDS patients, polygamists—all groups with oversexed reputations—from which I've read very boring diaries). Keep in mind that even the most sexually active diarists alive spend 95 percent of their lives in nonsexual activities—grocery shopping, cleaning, working, commuting. On a minute-to-minute basis? Dull.

The five diarists ahead lead five different lifestyles. Rather than getting lost in the details of who's sleeping with who—every nonmonogamous relationship is its own universe, and for many, the agreements and characters change on a monthly, if not weekly basis—it's much easier to understand these diarists from a priorities perspective. They are open to the idea that one person won't fulfill all their needs, and from there, they have each written an equation for their own lives, and filled in the appropriate variables. Which is a very different concept than promiscuity; some, in fact, are in closed relationships with more than one agreed upon lover. "Freedom" is the word The Corporate Gay Guy uses to describe his philosophy of sharing energy in whatever way makes sense, while committing wholeheartedly to his spouse.

Culturally, it's difficult to "see" these diarists' relationships. To their neighbors, all five appear to be monogamously married; more broadly speaking, they are cultural blank spots because mainstream media talks about sex in one of two contexts: traditional dating/marriage, or scandal. Imagine a morning television anchor announcing that last night he slept at his wife's, and tonight plans to sleep at Tamara's. He'd soon be a former television anchor. The result is that you've never read the honest tales of the diarists ahead, four parents who personally drop their kids at school in the morning, half of whom have graduate degrees, and all of whom have sex with other functional, tax-paying, consenting adults. This chapter fills in the blank spot.

Creative Relationships, Sexual and Not

Nonmonogamy is a solution that many diarists come to by experience, which is why these diarists skew older, averaging in their forties and beyond. These diarists mix and match relationship roles to fit their current needs, and add in sex where it mutually makes sense. They cherry pick. We begin with two dads who share parenting duties platonically: "While not romantically in love, we saw the practical advantages of sharing a household and having a child together," The Very Busy Gay Dad writes of his wife of twenty years. The Committed Corporate Gay Guy shares parenting duties with another couple.

None of the relationship structures and sexual behaviors ahead is remotely new—you have seen them all in the previous seven chapters. Structurally, The Busy Gay Dad is in a platonic Aspirer marriage (chapter 4). Behaviorally, The Corporate Gay Guy has found a committed life partner of ten years (chapter 4), while also continuing the same promiscuous behavior that bachelors display freely (chapter 1). It's only their combinations that raise eyebrows. But if you step back and think about these diarists' promiscuous pasts, suddenly committing to monogamy at age 34 would have been much more notable. They're consistent. Historically, The Very Busy Gay Dad's lifestyle (live-in wife, numerous hour-long lovers on the side) is not new either. Through the 19th century, ample evidence indicates that most lesbian and gay acts took place between people in heterosexual marriages, who didn't consider their acts to be an identity or lifestyle.

Nonmonogamous partners are nearly universally Lovers or Aspirers. Lovers are most common, because the lover urge for emotional and physical exploration dovetails nicely with nonmonogamy; Lovers also tend to enjoy examining emotion and jealousy. Aspirers make for excellent nonmonogamous partners when sexual freedom is one of the goals of the relationship, as is the case with The Porn Star Mom, or when the couple can achieve parenting and financial goals together. I have never seen a Partner open relationship, because it's incompatible with their sense of bodily co-ownership, as well as the stability and consistency on which Partners thrive.

For those uninitiated to gay male culture, both diaries ahead are eye-opening. Sex is readily available to The Corporate Committed Gay Guy, who cancels one date at 7:00 p.m., and hops in bed with a new Internet find by 10:00 p.m. Psychologists don't fuss over healthy promiscuity. As Ken Page, a Brooklyn psychotherapist, put it, "If a person can say that they feel emotionally fine during and after, and they have a life with a lot of love in it, who can call that bad?"

The Corporate, Committed Gay Guy
Enjoying Himself on a Work Trip

42, Chicago, Illinois

FRIDAY

7:15 a.m.: Wake up kinda of horny. Rub my boyfriend's butt a bit, but decide to hold back because he got home really late last night from a concert.

7:45 a.m.: Out of the shower. Don asks how babysitting went last night—we're coparenting a baby with a lesbian couple that lives nearby. He says he's taking the day off to do yard work. I have to work, but will come back for lunch.

11:00 a.m.: Don texts to ask what time I'm getting home. I wonder if he might have a tryst and wants to make sure I don't walk in on anything. We've been together for ten years, and its been open since day one, though we didn't act on that freedom until about a year in. We're very committed to each other, and emotionally extremely close.

12:30 p.m.: Workout, showering. Wondering if I should make sure I'm squeaky clean in case I have sex when I get home.

1:30 p.m.: Text with the mothers of our baby to see if they might want to join us for lunch. Don will be thrilled to see the baby.

1:45 p.m.: Preparing lunch. Don tells me that he met a young guy at a concert last night who said he was starting graduate school, and wants to start cleaning people's homes nude for $50 an hour. I ask if he's a prostitute. Don says he's not, then laughs and said that the guy texted earlier to ask if Don wanted him to come over for an estimate. We chuckle.

7:00 p.m.: Don and I are driving to see a play with Timothy, one of my oldest friends here—15 years now. Timothy always jokes that I've slept with whomever he's dating, and sure enough, he mentions yet another guy that I've slept with. Then he comments about a friend who has slept with Don. He's grossed out by the thought of my bf wanting someone so unattractive. I stay silent—it's Don's right to pick a fight if he wants. He doesn't.

8:30 p.m.: During the play, there's a section of interviews with gay men with HIV/AIDS. I obsess about Don with that guy. Earlier on, my fear of his getting infected—and a bit of machismo—made me suggest a rule that he wasn't allowed to have sex with others. Eventually, it seemed like a useless rule, so I gave it up. But it still worries me.

12:30 a.m.: Home. I tell Don that I'm bothered by the thought of him with that guy, but that I know I have no good case for it. He says he's glad I brought it up, because it had created tension between us all evening. He says he did it once, and also found the guy kind of gross after that. Still creepy, but I guess nothing can be done about it now.

SATURDAY

8:45 a.m.: Poking around Craigslist sex ads. Thinking a three-way might be fun. We'll see.

9:30 a.m.: A guy comes over, and we have a quick three-way. He was chubbier than I was expecting. But he was great at giving head, so I was happy.

5:00 p.m.: Shopping and prepping dinner while Don's out with a friend. Early on, we had to learn to manage our jealousy. That was good practice. We made some rules, including that we wouldn't do anything unsafe with someone else—neither of us has sex without a condom, or allows ejaculation in our mouths—and that if our actions became emotionally threatening to the other, we would stop right away. And we actively agreed to openness together, so while we might acknowledge some jealousy or hurt, we couldn't make the other one feel guilty for doing it.

7:00 p.m.: Horny, so I log into a porn site and beat off. While online, I see a hot video by a guy in New York. I email him to tell him I'm coming to town tomorrow, and ask if he'd be interested in blowing me while I'm there.

SUNDAY

7:00 a.m.: Wake up early. Don's making coffee, and we snuggle in the kitchen for a bit, and then do the dishes.

7:30 a.m.: Email from the New York guy. He says he lives in Chelsea, so we can hook up since I'll be staying in midtown. He wants to videotape him giving me head. Never been videotaped for a site. Would be kind of hot, I think.

7:31 a.m.: By the way, I met Don online. It was supposed to be a tawdry 20-minute hookup, but it lasted for 1.5 hours, and then we made a date to hookup again. And then three or four more times until Don said he was interested in more than just sex.

9:00 a.m.: Take the baby to Wiggleworms class, and then head to the airport. The baby's moms were friends of ours for three years, before they asked if we'd donate sperm for them to have a child. Don and I decided together that he'd be the donor. Two years or so after we all decided to do it, our baby was born.

6:00 p.m.: Fly to New York, and after checking into the hotel and walking around a bit, I text the Chelsea guy. He invites me over, and gives me a long, hot blowjob, which he films with a little video camera. The camera's intrusive, but also kind of fun. He says he'll have it up by the end of the day. He was pretty funny and nice.

10:30 p.m.: Having a couple of drinks with a friend I get together with when in New York. We actually met online abroad, when we were both there for work, and screwed around. More than that, though, it was cool to have someone to hang out with. We often see each other without having sex, but sometimes we do. When I'm away from home for a few days, it's a way of making emotional connections. I tell him that I'm tired and heading back to Manhattan. He's disappointed, and suggests that I come back to his place and he'll blow me.

11:00 p.m.: It's not hard to convince me. I decide to take a late taxi back to my hotel.

MONDAY

9:00 p.m.: Confirmed for tonight with a guy I'd talked to about hooking up with while I'm here. Full day of work.

7:00 p.m.: Guy emails that he's at a friend's place watching TV and will be late. I'm tired, tell him I'm gonna hit the sac.

9:15 p.m.: Mind wandering, horny. I'm putting an ad on Craigslist.

10:00 p.m.: Of the guys who answered, three were very hot. I told one to come over and he was hot, hot, hot. Both in looks and in bed. In his late 20s, Australian, moved to New York recently. We had sex for about 45 minutes, talked for about 15 minutes, and then I went to bed.

TUESDAY

7:37 a.m.: This is my final day here. I travel a lot, and I like it, but I also miss Don. We chat on the phone a couple of times a day. I wonder if my being gone for short bits of time helps us keep the attraction for each other alive.

9:00 a.m.: You're probably wondering what the purpose of sex is to me. In my relationship, earlier, it was about closeness and physical pleasure. Now it's also sometimes about adventure, usually three-way situations. Having sexual partners in the places where I visit is often a way of maintaining friendships in different places. It's either pleasure or seeking out something new. And the pleasure is typically in service of something else. It's a way of working out other things.

9:10 a.m.: And I know it sounds cheesy, but more than anything, it's a manifestation of freedom. I'm a person of color in largely white gay circles, where most gay men of color are reduced to stereotypes. It's often about negotiating racial complexities, and seeking freedom from them.

9:15 a.m.: The Internet has made sex a zillion times more available. I have less sex with my partner because it's so readily available with others. It's a slight release valve in that it makes our relationship work better, but it's also harmful in that it means our connection is sometimes interrupted by sex outside the relationship.

7:00 p.m.: Return home and Don is home from work. He looks kinda hot in his cycling shorts. We go upstairs and have sex, and then off to dinner.

9:00 p.m.: I told Don all about the Australian. Our agreement is that we have to be honest if asked, and earlier in our relationship, we used to ask a lot. Now, if something's particularly hot, I'll tell him. I told him that the Australian was cute, and had a huge uncircumcised cock.

WEDNESDAY

7:45 a.m.: It's a chilly morning. Wake up and spoon with Don for a bit.

8:30 p.m.: Don left before I did, and I was feeling frisky, so I jacked off to some Internet porn. Masturbation is almost always about release. It helps me clear my head, and puts me to sleep. I masturbate for about 2 minutes or so. As long as it takes me to come, and that's it. I usually want sex to last as long as possible.

5:30 p.m.: Ran home early so I could play with the baby a bit before baby bedtime (6:30). So I cooked, had a conference call, and played with the baby at the same time.

9:07 p.m.: A new friend named Benny also joined us all for dinner. He's recently divorced, and just moved. He's an extremely good looking guy, and has dated four women in the past two weeks. I ask him about his sex life. He says he rarely has sex before the third or fourth dates, and rarely initiates—the women usually do.

THURSDAY

7:30 a.m.: Typical morning. Five or ten minutes in bed spooning, then get ready.

10:00 a.m.: A colleague is in my office. Her husband is an alcoholic who had delirium tremens the last time he tried to sober up. He's in rehab, and she's committed to staying with him and seeing it all through.

10:15 a.m.: I am incredibly moved by the conversation. I am struck that they're learning so much through this process. She ends by saying that it's such a shame that people who are so close never really talk to each other.

11:00 a.m.: Thinking about therapy. I went into therapy when I first met Don. We broke up a zillion times the first year. I thought I wanted to be in a relationship but I also sensed it meant the end of my freedom, and I tied that freedom to my development as a human being. In 1.5 years of therapy, I practiced having discussions with my therapist that I was afraid would hurt Don. I realized that things couldn't work out if I didn't raise them, and that the things I thought would be really scary to Don weren't.

8:50 p.m.: Reading in bed. Don and I barely have any tastes in common, like reading or music or politics. It freaked me out for a while. Then I realized two things simultaneously: I was afraid of having a committed relationship, because "forever" is scary, and that the things that are important to share is a commitment to communication, and making what is important to the other person important to you. Once I dealt with those two issues, everything's been good.

· · · · · · · · · · · · · · · · · **Diary Insight** · · · · · · · · · · · · · · · ·

These two diarists are master communicators. In a week of many lovers, The Corporate Gay Guy has less drama with his spouse than many monogamous couples ignite in a single meal. Watch as The Very Busy Gay Dad states to his lovers exactly what he wants to happen in the next 30 minutes.

· ·

The Very Busy Gay Dad Married to His Kid's Mother

46, Oakland County, Missouri

MONDAY

7:44 a.m.: In bed, receive notice of six new Twitter followers. Three of them have naked torsos as their user photo. I accept them all. My one real email is from my best friend, Todd, who tells me he's broken up with his boyfriend of four years. Think of a reply while I cuddle my spouse.

8:35 a.m.: Write Todd a quick email to say how sorry I am. Despite being sworn to secrecy, I tell my wife. She's not surprised.

8:40 a.m.: The summary: I'm a technically bisexual, emotionally gay man, who's married. While not romantically in love, we saw the practical advantages of sharing a household and having a child together. My spouse knew of my sexuality when we met, and most of our eighteen years together have been in an open relationship. It works for us, though we tend to keep our sexual lives separate. I work at home as a writer, so my time is my own.

1:38 p.m.: The wife came home for lunch, which was both pleasant and unusual. We sat on the sofa while watching the Food Network.

Mid-lunch, my partnered play buddy Jon emailed to see if I was available. I wrote no, but check back later in the week.

2:18 p.m.: A 22-year-old named Beck from North Carolina wrote to tell me that he reads my blog and is inspired because we both have southern roots, and he dreams of a life in which he doesn't hide his sexuality. I'm more than a little touched.

4:41 p.m.: Our teenager overhears us on the Todd breakup issue, and weighs in: "His boyfriend was pretty shitty anyway." Can't disagree.

5:06 p.m.: My wife and I hug for a couple of minutes. Then she asks me to sniff her armpits to check her new deodorant. This is two decades of marriage: the sweet and the practical.

6:09 p.m.: My mailbox is full of sex offers for tonight, although I haven't logged into a sex site all day. Only one is from a guy I've met before—a police officer. I can't stand the guy. I've got theater plans anyway.

7:59 p.m.: We're the only male-female couple in the audience. It's a Charles Busch play, and the central character is in drag. A man next to me is totally my type—lean, scruffy, twenties, and covered with amazing tattoos. When he pulls out his iPhone, I lean over to perhaps catch his name. My wife asks, "Reading anything interesting?" She rolls her eyes. Giggling.

10:27 p.m.: Another email from the 22 year-old, full of flattery, and an email from my lover in Kentucky, which I'll save for tomorrow.

TUESDAY

9:35 a.m.: I like my hairdresser because he gives $40 haircuts for $10. We met on a gay bowling team. Throughout the cut he keeps up a stream of profanity, racial epithets, and sex talk.

9:45 a.m.: Most gay guys translate "bisexual" to mean that I never fool around with other women. He seems to think I do nothing but. "You got it comin' out of your ears, pussy hound! Don't ya? All in and out of pussy, all the damned time, like an OB-GYN." Right. Exactly.

10:10 a.m.: Jon writes to ask if I could do him today. Sure.

11:00 a.m.: Wife home unexpectedly, announcing that she doesn't have school this afternoon. Cancel with Jon. One of our long-standing courtesies is that neither has sexual partners to the house when anyone else is there.

11:10 a.m.: Wife appears with her bag and announces that she's going in anyway. I'm so confused.

11:42 a.m.: Replying to my lover in Kentucky, Bill. We met through my blog, and began corresponding about books, southern culture, and cooking. Then I visited him during a visit to my Dad's. It was a sweet night of lovemaking and talking. Bill engages my intellect more than most, which makes me carve out a daily place for him. Though it's merely email, it's as if I'm gossiping with a lover over coffee.

12:54 p.m.: For the first time since Friday (Saturday?) I masturbate. I don't usually look at porn. I'd much rather enjoy thinking about someone I've been with and what we did. Today my thoughts bounced between Bill and Beck's photo.

2:13 p.m.: My back fence neighbor is always vaguely flirty. Today he decided it was time to remove his shirt and point his chest in my direction. "Feast your eyes!" he yelled, I think to catch my attention . . . though ostensibly to his wife, who stood two feet away.

5:00 p.m.: Lying in bed, and my wife is cracking her toes against my shin while venting about how all her students are mentally checked out for the summer.

5:05 p.m.: I ask my wife if she'd marry me all over again. "Of course. We have a great life. And we went into it with eyes wide open, which is more than most of those poor souls."

7:35 p.m.: Took wife to dinner to cheer her. I feel safe in my relationship. We both firmly believe that people drift in and out of our lives, and we have the potential to form lasting friendships and relationships. I have a friend as my spouse, and someone who respects a career that isn't exactly making riches. I have a roof over my head. These are all good things.

WEDNESDAY

7:38 a.m.: Five new Twitter followers. Three naked torsos this time, two faces. Three blog fans have sent me unsolicited photos. They emerge from the anonymity of readers and establish a foothold in my imagination.

9:30 a.m.: Browsing Craigslist Missed Connections. Every ad reads to me like a little prayer of "Dear God, please let me have been noticed."

11:46 a.m.: Two emails, five minutes apart, from men wanting sex today. One is a 20-year-old art student who's been wanting to sketch and get naked with me; the other is Jon.

11:48 a.m.: Jon will be here at noon.

12:15p.m.: The sex is perfunctory: we kissed, he sucked me, and then I did him. Once we were done, he zipped up, clapped me on the back, and left. Sex with Jon is always regrettably brief because his boyfriend is afraid he's cheating, and keeps him on a tight leash. The boyfriend is right to be suspicious.

7:16 p.m.: Preparing one of my wife's favorite dinners, and the sight of little tubs of hummus (which she loves) and strawberries bring an enormous smile to her face. Does the trade-off between perfect sexual compatibility and thoughtfulness make me a good mate?

9:52 p.m.: Beck sends a chat invite. I login and am greeted with an invitation to view him on camera. His ultraconservative religious parents are watching *American Idol* downstairs, while he removes his clothes in a slow striptease and masturbates himself to climax. I simply watch and appreciate, and then chat with him about his graduate school plans. What a polite, articulate, and sweet kid—with a slamming body.

THURSDAY

7:26 a.m.: Two emails from blog readers demanding to know why I'm gay and married. I politely thank them for reading—I generally don't feel an obligation to explain or justify my relationship.

7:49 a.m.: Facebook dilemma over Todd's ex. In olden days, you simply didn't see the ex much anymore. On Facebook or on Twitter, do you drop them? Ignore them?

8:52 a.m.: A guy I occasionally have sex with emails. This particular gentleman—my age, a white-collar professional—enjoys taking an afternoon off of work, renting a room in a cheap motel in the worst part of the city, and having guy after guy over. I went to one of his parties once, but found myself put off by both the seediness of the room and of the guys trooping in and out. I gave today's invitation a polite pass.

3:37 p.m.: Beck is online. Our southern backgrounds are remarkably similar, but I feel extremely fortunate to have had liberal-crusader parents with hippie tendencies. My mother provided dire threats not to marry any girls until I'd lived with them for at least a year in order to determine our sexual compatibility.

3:42 p.m.: My wife discreetly inquires of my evening plans, which I interpret to mean she wants a dalliance of her own. We don't ask each other for details, usually. I know she's been seeing a guy who is cheating on his wife, and he believes her to be cheating as well.

8:45 p.m.: Our best friends of a decade live down the street—a gay couple. They pick me up and take me to a gay bar.

11:30 p.m.: My wife comes in, clutching her bag and looking pretty. I asked how her evening was. "Eh," she replies. We both tend to be private.

12:30 a.m.: Despite the warm evening, I'm falling asleep with her spooned up against me.

FRIDAY

9:30 a.m.: One of my regular playmates just called, asking if I could come over. If a daytime opportunity arises to have a little playtime, I usually can take it. I worked a lot yesterday.

1:00 p.m.: Just leaving my playmate's house. He's all of 20; I met him online. He enjoys being naked and alone in his bed, and for me to enter his apartment, find him in the dark bedroom, and strip down to crawl into bed with him. I enjoyed making slow love to him today, as I usually do. We made out, I stroked him until he purred, slowly and deliberately. He always calls me "daddy." A lot of the young guys do. I used to resent it, and thought it was a reflection on my age. But now I think it's more my dominance and assertiveness. These young guys mostly want to be led, and shepherded, and praised when they do a good job.

1:04 p.m.: I do wish I had the courage to explore my submissive side. Taking the passive role in anal intercourse doesn't come

naturally. I find the loss of control a little frightening. I also sometimes have secret rape fantasies. I was raped in my early twenties—I
met my spouse in a rape survivors' group session, in fact—which is
why I have no wish to trivialize the seriousness of a violent act with
a fantasy that's less about violence and more about surrendering
control.

2:30 p.m.: Chili's for late lunch with my wife, listening to a couple
at an adjacent table, arguing. They're sniping, hissing vicious threats
and accusations. Wife looks upset, so I (the guy who gets to kill spiders
and shush loud movie talkers) suggest that they keep their voices
down. In return, I am told to mind my own business.

10:09 p.m.: Tonight we sat on our back deck as a family and played
board games. I intend to avenge my spectacular losses tomorrow as a
Guitar Hero drummer.

SATURDAY

1:03 p.m.: While I power-wash the deck off the back of my house,
my backyard neighbor watches from a lawn chair pointed in my direction. For his benefit, I unbutton my shirt. He nods at me, and when
I'm done, goes indoors. Flirty bastard.

1:04 p.m.: I'm referring to both of us, I suppose.

5:04 p.m.: At a birthday barbecue party. I suppose it's a Republican's nightmare get-together: The hosts are a gay couple, and one of
their fathers is here with his fifth wife, and the young children from his
fourth marriage. Our gay best friends are here, as are a pair of long-
married lesbians, a bisexual single mother and her two kids, and one
lone traditional straight couple. It's a good group.

8:51 p.m.: My wife and the married straight guy are in a spirited
debate over don't-ask-don't-tell. Quoth the straight guy: 'They're all
so worried some gay guy is gonna suck them while they sleep! I was
in the military for eighteen years and I gotta tell you, I never got so
lucky!"

11:10 p.m.: Everyone leaves stuffed and more than slightly toasted.

11:16 p.m.: Lying in bed with my spouse. It's been a typical week—
the usual mixture of domestic affection and extramarital sex. Though
the road we've followed isn't perhaps for everyone

SUNDAY

8:43 a.m.: Such a nice warm, quiet Sunday. My wife and kid are off ushering at church, leaving me utterly alone.

11:10 a.m.: At a buddy's house. We've been casual sex partners for over a year—long enough that I don't really remember how we met. We begin making out immediately, barely stopping as we strip and fall onto the sofa. After some mutual oral sex, I do him as he masturbates furiously to some porn. I prefer to attend to matters at hand. I shut out the distraction, climax, and return home after some small talk.

2:52 p.m.: When it rains, it pours. Invitation to meet an out-of-town businessman stranded in a hotel. Though he's attractive as hell, I instead delight my wife by cleaning the deck for summer.

4:41 p.m.: At the supermarket for the weekly grocery run. It's my turn to pay. I pull out a $50 gift card. My wife raises her eyebrows. Two months ago, a gay guy in a sexless relationship paid me $200 in supermarket gift cards to simply watch me masturbate. My wife snorts.

5:41 p.m.: This sex diary reminds me how I'm not accustomed to talking about my home life, work life, and private life in one place. Short as these entries may be, they represent my everyday life more fully. Confirms what I've always suspected—that a lot of us don't fit into the rigid little cubbyholes that we, as a society, tend to create for sexual roles. I think more of us are odd parcels and undeliverable mail than we assume. ✱✱✱

A Brief History of Open Relationships

When I first began editing diaries, it was tricky for me to grasp the various shapes of open relationships. I wasn't used to them. Americans don't do well with ambiguity. We like rules and clarity; we describe people as the "current boyfriend" or the "ex," and lack terms for the in-between. Breakups make sense to us. But The Corporate Committed Gay Guy regularly interacts with a dozen sometime-lovers. Open diarists' lives are commonly devoid of breakups, because there's rarely a reason to formally cut ties. And their side relationships don't necessarily *go* anywhere—The

Very Busy Gay Dad has lots of lovers whom he sees a few times a year, and that's it. There are no absolutes; only moving around and readjusting to fit the couple's agreements, and the diarist's current needs.

I asked Helen Fisher for her take on open relationships. She pointed out that people in open relationships tend to enjoy the intense, early stages of love, as well as transparency and communication. "Theoretically speaking, it's very grown up. The problem is that the human animal is not built to openly share. We are a jealous creature. So you may have fun on Saturday, but will spend Monday through Thursday talking about jealousy and hurt feelings. But if you are built to share, you can build the kind of marriage that you want to." Which is precisely what the diarists ahead have done.

She notes that open mating has been around much longer than closed mating. Prehistoric humans were not possessive; food, land, and children weren't "owned" in preagricultural society, so neither were mates. The sense of mate ownership appeared only after the rise of land and property ownership. Cacilda Jetha and Christopher Ryan's book *Sex at Dawn* explicates this anthropological history. As he told *Salon*, "Human sexuality is distorted by our modern conception of marriage. This insistence that love and sex always go together is erroneous . . . The American insistence on mixing love and sex, and expecting passion to last forever, is leading to great suffering that is tragic and unnecessary."[1] As you've gathered, open relationships are rather popular among the social sciences set.

There is a strong anthropological argument that some humans are evolutionarily designed to be less than monogamous. Ryan's book outlines many theories, the most cocktail-worthy of which is the Testicle Theory: that animals with enormous testicles, such as bonobos and chimpanzees, are nonmonogamous, and use their large equipment to essentially rocket-launch sperm into the uterus, beating out other recent visitors. Monogamous animals like gorillas and gibbons have tiny testicles. Human testicles are comparatively large, but not quite bonobo-size, which, according to the theory, renders them designed to be semimonogamous. Biologists also like to point out that fidelity is rare in nature: Over 95 percent of mammals have multiple sex partners. This is not the strongest argument, because animals also do things such as eating their young and walk in front of traffic. More convincing is that the many men with a gene that regulates vasopressin—a cuddle hormone—are more likely to stray.[2]

A Few Contextual Notes: Fifteen percent of adults enjoy half of all sexual encounters. Many of them are in this chapter. And yet much of the sex itself is vanilla. Their relationships are nontraditional; their beds, for the most part, are conventional. The exception is The Kink-Lifestyle Dad who is simply not fulfilled by vanilla sex. When I first began editing the diaries, I had no idea why seemingly happy, balanced diarists would elevate kinky sexuality to account for large portions of their private and public lives. "I am drawn to more intense kinds of sexual experiences than others," writes The Kink-Lifestyle Dad, who spent the first twenty years of his adult life in monogamous relationships with vanilla sex. "Things like BDSM and bondage I like a lot, and sensation play. I enjoy sexual contact that is much more intentional and where the connection is much more powerful." It makes him feel whole.

Much of the S&M we see in mainstream culture is not S&M at all. It's vanilla sex with handcuffs. Or a rope. Different. Two key, nonintuitive understandings helped me understand kink and S&M: First, kink and S&M are often surprisingly intellectual. The arousal is usually the result of embarrassment (psychological stress) or controlled pain. As The Kink-Lifestyle Dad explains, his sex life is mostly psychological, and intercourse is not necessarily part of every sexual act. The idea is to create "scenes," often involving preplanned role-playing, in which much of the turn-on is feeling powerful or vulnerable, by pushing psychological boundaries and/ or sexualizing typical household items that aren't usually sexualized. In short, it's a mind fuck, and scenes can go on for hours and hours. And second, scenes and S&M are largely about endorphins. Physical orgasms and lovey-dovey cuddling drive most of the vanilla sex in this book; the kink play dates of The Kink-Lifestyle Dad and his wife are a matter of inducing a natural, extended endorphin high.

Yep. They're high.

Psychologists are quite supportive of fetishes and kink. "Fetishes are all in the head," says psychoanalyst Dr. David Greenan. "When we develop fetishes, what we're talking about is sense memory. These are early feelings of being aroused and being sensual. In adulthood, the person is trying to replicate those earliest experiences of arousal. And it's fine, as long as it feels comfortable for the couple and doesn't get in their way of relating to one another."

The Kink-Lifestyle Dad mentions a couple of scenes of violence. Fantasies involving violence are exceedingly common in the diaries. The British Sexual Fantasy Research Project, a study of 19,000 British fantasies, found that "many fantasies contain strong imagery of sadism, masochism and other forms of harm. If any of us could manage to put many of our more aggressive fantasies into practice, we would end up in prison." The Kink-Lifestyle Dad emphasizes that his scenes are intricately planned out, complete with safe words and safe sex (condoms, gloves), and that the motto of the S&M community is "safe, sane, and consensual."

What always strikes me in this chapter—beyond the responsible, constant condom use—is just how well these diarists know themselves. They are deeply self-analyzed, with no closets left unexplored. They have to be, in order to state precisely what they'd like to happen, and to set clear boundaries—which require knowing exactly what they want, a skill rare among the diarists in this book.

I've long joked that this book should be called "the options," presenting the relationships and options that people are *actually* choosing—a panacea to a world where so much of our understanding of relationships are inaccurately defined from the outside. We begin the adventure on a rare sunny morning in Seattle.

The Kink-Lifestyle Dad

45, Seattle, Washington

SATURDAY

10:00 a.m.: Starting late. Morning lovemaking with Alison, my wife of just over a year.

12:00 p.m.: We're at a holistic peer counseling retreat. I've done the training before, and Alison wanted to do it because the counseling tools are really useful in a lot of situations: how to be an active listener, how to pay attention in a focused way. We use it in the context of doing scenes, or tantric tantras, or sex priestessing.

8:00 p.m.: About to do nonorgasmic sex with Alison. I enjoy it pretty frequently, I'd say a couple of times a week. It's basically a lot of sensual play without any real direction. The intention isn't "oh, let's go have sex." It involves a lot of making out, massage, and can involve penetrative sex. The point is just to play and be with each other.

10:00 p.m.: Two hours of delicious, nonorgasmic sex. Though not intended, Alison had a very powerful orgasm. It's an amazing feeling to be in that state of connectedness and intimacy, orgasmic or not.

SUNDAY

9:00 a.m.: Woke up thinking of Jennifer. I haven't seen her for over a month, and recently talked to her on the phone. I miss her. Introductions: Alison is my wife. We have been married for just over a year. We are polyamorous, and have dated many other people since we first met four years ago. Jennifer is my lover who lives in a nearby city. We met at the end of last year at a party in her city. She is also in a committed relationship with a primary partner, and has several other lovers.

12:00 p.m.: Second day of peer counseling class. It's nice to have someone hear whatever you want to express for a period, and then switch places.

6:49 p.m.: I am a bit exhausted and frustrated. Alison has dates the next two evenings and I don't, which makes it more difficult. Either I can push to get the personal space that I need tonight, or try to wait until tomorrow when I will be on my own anyway. Bleh.

8:00 p.m.: We were going to do a knife play scene, where I would use a knife to threaten her and cut off her clothes. Scenes like that bring up a lot of emotions and issues. And that's why it's hot—you bring up more of a psychological and emotional connection. We decided not to do it, because I was feeling pretty volatile. My experience is, if you're feeling volatile, don't do scenes where there's something potentially dangerous involved. Cuddling.

11:00 p.m.: Alison and I just had a long talk. We've been running into some issues around codependency, and being individuals in our relationship. We talked about respecting and creating our own boundaries for nearly three hours.

MONDAY

8:00 a.m.: Client meeting. I usually run my practice from home, but am out of the house all day today.

1:15 p.m.: Take a break to look up knot ties for a suspension we're doing this week that is, from an engineering perspective, extravagant and challenging. As you have probably gathered, I am drawn to more intense kinds of sexual experiences than others. I like things like BDSM and bondage, and sensation play. I've studied tantra practices, which are more intense ways of connecting around sexual energy. I enjoy sexual contact that is much more intentional, and where connection is much more powerful.

4:00 p.m.: Alison and I haven't crossed paths yet, and I didn't cross paths with anyone other than clients today. That's not very sexy.

5:00 p.m.: Called Alison and told her to have fun on her date. The guy wants to do a cock-and-ball torture scene, where she'll kick and punch him. (There are ways you can do it safely. Namely, swinging upward, so the scrotum has space to move.) For me, it would be unpleasant, but there are people to whom this is a very big turn-on. The purpose is for Alison to experience doing this sort of thing (she's never done it before), and to be coached by someone who really enjoys it, and see if it's something she wants to pursue.

8:00 p.m.: Home. I originally thought about trying to arrange a date, but I just didn't get off my butt to do it. Instead I went shopping, and meandered around in that *I don't have anything better to do* kind of way. I bought food.

8:30 p.m.: Called my daughter. I have a child who lives primarily with her mother, but spends summers with me. I have established very solid boundaries between her and my private life, primarily that what I do is not open for examination. This said, she knows that we are intimate outside our marriage. I do not show her the toys or tools I might take on a date, nor does she know that we might be having an explicitly sexual portion. When she asks for it, any general information she wants is readily available. I've never dated anyone that I wouldn't want her to meet. I've been decorating her room for the summer, and we talked about the colors.

12:30 a.m.: Alison's home. We cuddled and checked in. Pillow talking about how it went and the basics of what went on. My sense is that she came away from it kind of neutral, not really rushing out the door to do it again, but also that she had a good time.

TUESDAY

9:00 a.m.: I got up, ate breakfast, and am working. Alison is sleeping in.

11:00 a.m.: So during the course of most days, I email and text with a number of people who I'm either playing with or interested in playing with. I use a couple of adult social networking websites, and Facebook. I don't really think of it as separate from my life—I'll be on Facebook and I'll send someone an email saying how much I like the photo they put up of themselves in a corset, the same way I comment if I like their new kitten.

11:15 a.m.: Emailing a potential partner who is new to this. I too am fairly new—I was married to my daughter's mother in a long-term monogamous relationship. And before that, I searched for people I could have orgasms with. After the divorce, I started educating myself on the spectrum of sexual experiences, which led me more into BDSM and sex magik and tantra, and in the process of encountering those things, started to realize that sex really was a divine act. At first my quest was about kink and creating new and interesting sensations and getting off. Now it's about having experiences where orgasm is a possibility, but not an inevitability.

7:30 p.m.: Alison left for a date with a friend of hers. This is more of a bondage date. This particular guy doesn't enjoy more traditional sexual experiences—he doesn't enjoy kissing, and doesn't crave penetrative sex. All of his arousal comes from being restrained. He has quite a collection of bondage equipment, and Alison puts him into the equipment. He's under a lot of it, so their interaction is more like dry humping. Nonpenetrative. She really has fun with this guy. It's a playful thing they have. While the ball kicking guy was all about an experience, this one is about their friendship together.

9:36 p.m.: Tonight, it's nice to just lie about and watch a not-so-great movie. Brief visit by Cat was a nice interruption and brought me out of a bit of a stupor. She gave me a wonderful hug before she left that woke up my skin a little. Cat is a former lover of both Alison and mine who is probably our closest friend.

10:21 p.m.: A little bored. Alison's having more dates than I am this week, but in other stretches, I've had more. Went online to Second Life and talked to a few people I had met before, which was unsatisfying but okay. Will watch some porn and then maybe sleep.

WEDNESDAY

7:30 a.m.: Morning sex with Alison. She got aroused, but hadn't had any orgasms last night or Monday night. So we rolled around with toys.

8:30 a.m.: Getting started a bit slowly this morning. I have a date later to do yoni massage and I am excited about that. I will need to get myself going but I have time. I also have caffeine.

10:00 a.m.: Preparing my "kit" for the date. Our agreement is that we use barriers (gloves, condoms, dental dams) for any sort of penetrative contact with any of our partners, or oral contact other than kissing. So I'm restocking my blue nitrile gloves.

4:00 p.m.: Had a fifth appointment with an older woman who's had past sexual trauma. We do sacred intimate work. Basically I'll do vaginal or yoni massage with her and the goal has nothing to do with my pleasure or my arousal. I'm helping her explore touch, and different ways of being touched, and expressing where she likes and doesn't like to be touched. She wants to get past her own fear of interacting sexually with men, and has complete control in a nonthreatening way.

6:00 p.m.: Rushing to make up for the time away from my desk.

THURSDAY

11:00 a.m.: Alison and I played like bunnies all morning, which was unexpected. We were in bed making out and playing for the first hour, and having sex for the second. Alison is not particularly quick to orgasm, and neither am I in most cases.

12:00 p.m.: Body's tired. We finished up with a quasi role-play. It was a dominant-submissive interaction where I was dominant, and pushing her to suck my cock and open herself up to me, being penetrated with my fingers. The kind of sex we did coming out of that was much harder, much more physically aggressive, and a pretty forceful workout. We did a lot of positions, and ended in doggie style with her using a magic wand vibrator to orgasm.

4:58 p.m.: Alison's been depressed and moody all day and I am really not in the mood to do the suspension we're planning for tonight.

8:15 p.m.: We just had a couples counseling session. It was a dumb idea to do counseling and then try to do an intense scene. The counseling brought up some stuff around our enmeshment and poor barrier management, and it was very emotional. This said, it's hard to blame the situation between Alison and I as "her problem" when it shows up in my other relationships as well.

9:00 p.m.: The scene's not happening. We were going to do a fairly elaborate suspension, which requires focus and not screwing it up, because it's an inverted suspension from her waist and leg, and she can fall on her head. It's one we've talked about doing for a long time.

10:47 p.m.: Just stepping out to talk to Lise, a friend planning Alison's birthday gift. We're going to do a gangbang scene. No, it's not a surprise. You can't really surprise someone with something like that. I asked my friend to help because I don't know many guys who have the skills to do it. She knows more guys than I do, and their sexual histories and capabilities.

12:00 a.m.: Just got back. Lise is confident that she can pull together a group of guys who are careful. Alison and I have talked about doing this for a while. Anyone can get a dick hard and come in a room and do somebody—that would be fairly easy to arrange. But I don't want Alison to catch any STIs out of it, and if the scene becomes too emotionally intense, we want them to back off and care for Alison. I don't know many who are capable of pulling that off. Gang rape by people who care for you is important.

1:15 a.m.: We're sleeping separately tonight, because it's been a wacky day.

FRIDAY

6:30 a.m.: Up early to clean the house. We're hosting a third and final sex magik workshop this weekend. For a few years I've been doing sex magik events called Aphrodite Temples, where you create a multi-day spiritual context for people to have sexual experiences in. At a certain point you lose track of goals and time, and begin to encounter sex as a spiritual thing. It's like a long meditation.

2:00 p.m.: Traveling for a client meeting most of the day.

5:00 p.m.: In my car, waiting to see Lise again, this time with Alison. This scene has been challenging for me because Alison is not interested in having me in the room with her when it's going on. And I'm not that interested in being in the room. My role in the scene is to first make it happen, then step back and let it happen, and when it's over, come back in with Alison and be there to support her and process the emotional aftereffects. So what I get, in many ways, is a closer connection to her, a deeper kind of intimacy that includes an experience that's very challenging for her. It means we're really there for each other.

6:00 p.m.: Lise is talking with Alison alone, about what emotions it's bringing up. I'm feeling good—I get to facilitate a fantasy for someone who I love on a very deep level. And she gets to have a really hot fantasy.

11:45 p.m.: We're at a party together. Alison wandered away and made out with a couple of different people at the party. Just playing—I'm fairly sure her intention isn't to go somewhere and have penetrative sex and orgasms. And I just finished a negotiation with a friend I'm going to play with Wednesday. It wasn't what a lot of people would consider a sexual situation. It was more like, "Do you like being touched like this? Do you like hair pulling?" I love my life. I have really smart, hot lovers. The beauty of polyamory is that I can allow myself to expand as deeply into my relationships as I desire.

The Porn Star Mom Who Is Feeling Insecure This Week

38, Las Vegas, Nevada

MONDAY

5:00 a.m.: Husband woke up first. I peeked at his butt as he headed to the bathroom. He had that morning hard-on guys always get. I love a pre-pee penis. Sometimes I get to him before he can get out of bed, but not this morning.

5:15 a.m.: He brings me coffee. He does this every morning.

6:30 a.m.: Answering emails. I get 50–75 a day from fans. Most are tame. A few guys want sex, and a couple blowjob requests. I don't mind them asking, but I like when they get a little more descriptive because that turns me on.

9:00 a.m.: Pilates, and drop the little man off at school. Big kiss for little man.

9:15 a.m.: Home, studying dialogue. Dev—that's my husband—is explaining the promo we're shooting this afternoon. I'm gonna be in a big Jacuzzi tub with my girlfriend Rachel, and we're going to try to get guys to sign up to win a date with us. I love Rachel and I'm kind of excited about taking a sudsy soak with her.

12:00 p.m.: They don't have a makeup artist for this, but I've got it down to a science. Have to shave my legs too. I'm kind of horny. I'm horny a lot. I tell Dev that we could do a quickie if he wants, but his brain is all about work, so he isn't into it. Usually I'd just use my vibrator, but I know I'm going to have fun with Rachel soon anyway.

12:45 p.m.: Crew arrives. They're in my bathroom setting up cameras and lights, and I'm applying makeup. Naked, of course. I love being naked in front of people. I ask if they mind, and they don't. It's a turn-on because in the mirror, I can see them peeking over at me. Dev loves it. He doesn't get jealous of my character Sunset—he loves the attention she always gets.

1:15 p.m.: Rachel is here. She's brought a little bottle of vodka and I have cranberry juice. Dev makes us a cocktail to loosen us up. The script is really simple, but I always manage to mess up my lines. I think too hard. Rachel is much better.

2:00 p.m.: In the hot, soapy tub, lathering each others' boobies. Everyone is crowding around, even Dev. The director feeds us our lines and, of course, I mess up. Over and over again. Rachel gets her stuff perfect. But my mess ups have everyone laughing (except Dev, who takes everything seriously).

3:15 p.m.: If we were at a porn shoot we'd be having sex, but it's a wrap. Dev leaves to pick up our son. The house is empty except for Rachel and I, so we've got 15 minutes before the boys get back. I'm all over Rachel. I love to kiss pussy, and she lets me. I know I won't have a chance to get off, but I don't care. I just want to kiss Rachel's sweet coochie and make her orgasm, and by the way she wiggles, I know I'm doing a good job.

8:30 p.m.: All the domestic stuff is done—homework, dinner, etc. Dev and I are in bed. People think that because of what I do and living in Vegas, that I'm up late. Actually, we try to get to bed before nine every night.

8:45 p.m.: It doesn't take much effort to get Dev aroused. Of course, he knows I'm really horny, and he doesn't want to do any work. So after getting him real hard with my mouth I climb on top of his body and do all the driving. Guys love a girl on top because it's such an awesome view. I'm straddling him and pounding away and his hands are getting busy—playing with my boobies and pulling my hair (I love when my hair is pulled, not too hard, but just enough). I come before he pops. I sleep so well that I don't care about the *Law & Order* reruns.

TUESDAY

4:40 a.m.: Dev's got his erection in the crack of my butt and I grind a little, but he's just teasing. His mind is already on his day. He thinks too much!

6:15 a.m.: Coffee, email. Today I've got some naughty emails! One is from a young'un in Paris, 20 years old. She's a big fan, and I like to flirt with her. Another guy writes love poems. I don't mind these guys being in love and such, but it's a little weird, and it's not much of a turn-on.

6:25 a.m.: Email: "I want to bend you over and spank your hot ass and pull your hair and screw you from behind." Now, that's what I like!

11:00 a.m.: Tuesday business lunch date with Dev. We sit in our usual seats, and Dev and his associate talk. There's always at least one fan asking for my autograph. I carry movies and 8x10s with me.

12:23 p.m.: A guy at the bar has a t-shirt for me. It's become a running gag, since the general manager once gave me a shirt, and I tried it on, on the spot (no bra). So now everyone loves to bring me t-shirts. The cell phones are clicking away. I'm a total exhibitionist.

1:00 p.m.: Bathroom break. Dev always walks me to the bathroom when we're in public, just in case.

9:25 p.m.: We're in bed and Dev is making love to me. He's on top and he's being sweet and slow and I'm really getting into it. And then his cell phone rings. I say, "You are *not* going to answer that!" But Dev lives with his stupid phone—he says you never know when it could be important.

9:27 p.m.: Now, my web site has a contact number for me, but it's Dev's number, so he can screen calls. And fans call at all hours and Dev is forever answering. And this time he's smirking at me and actually talking to the guy. He tells the guy that he's in luck, that I just so happen to be available. He doesn't pull out. He's such an asshole sometimes, and he hands me the phone. I'm pissed but I decide to have a little fun.

9:32 p.m.: I push Dev off me and crawl on top of him. I mount him and begin to talk dirty to the fan. The guy loves it, of course, and when I ask him what he'd do to me if I were with him right now, he gets into it. And so there I am doing my old man while talking dirty to this fan and it's a total turn-on and I can tell Dev is digging it too. And who knows? Maybe all three of us got off.

9:43 p.m.: I place the phone back on Dev's nightstand and tell him he's bisexual, because we just had a three-way with another guy. "Whatever, Mariane."

WEDNESDAY

6:05 a.m.: Dev plunks on the bed beside me with coffee, and he's rambling. I need that coffee and I need him to shut up. Burying head beneath pillows.

6:15 a.m.: Dev has a big announcement. He's been brokering a deal for me to be in an indie film, playing myself, and I guess it went through. It's a fair price for me to play myself, and it's mainstream. I'm excited.

7:00 a.m.: I don't care about emails. I'd rather sit and talk with my son while he eats breakfast. Dev will rant, but tough.

11:00 a.m.: It's my day off, and we're at the bar feeding twenty dollar bills into the video poker machines. Dev is telling the bartender about the movie and about my gig at the Hard Rock on Friday—he's such a promoter. I lose on purpose just so I can move to another machine across the bar, away from him. Don't get me wrong. I love my husband, but he's always in work mode.

3:00 p.m.: I'm in the guest room, to get away from the TV and the lights Dev keeps on. He walks in. He knows what I'm up to because my hands are under the covers. I'm masturbating with the little red vibrator. He smiles, shakes his head and I say, "What?" And I could shoot him because I almost came and he ruined it!

8:30 p.m.: We're in bed. There is no sexual energy here. We're not mad or anything, it's just not a sexual night.

12:45 a.m.: My stepchild bursts into our room yelling at her dad that he deleted her important college math stuff. I wake up pissed, but I know better than to get involved. She slams our door and then bangs around, making a lot of noise. He doesn't want to talk about it.

THURSDAY

6:45 a.m.: Email from Greg. He's an average-looking, very overweight sweetheart who is an unpaid mascot for a sports team and he saves his money for visits to me because he doesn't have female company otherwise. He booked this date a month ago, and I forgot. No biggie though. I'll call him in a few hours and see him tonight.

7:30 p.m.: I'm getting dolled up. I don't dress quite as flashy as I would if going to, say, the Palazzo or Bellagio. I hate looking like a total hooker, but I get recognized—a lot—and I don't want to look average either.

8:30 p.m.: I'm heading off to the Golden Nugget. I call Greg from the car. He's really excited, and I'm excited because in reality, I love what I do. I love the attention and I love providing company, especially to the kind of guys who don't get much loving from hot chicks.

8:55 p.m.: Greg is such a sweetheart. He's a big boy—must be about 300 pounds, in a pullover shirt with a collar and clean jeans. I give him a big kiss. Why? A lot of eyes are on us, and kissing him on the mouth makes him proud. We have a few drinks at the bar—I'm never in a rush with my guys. It's not that boom-boom-boom thing with me. I hate that. It seems cheap and unfair.

9:40 p.m.: Now we're in his room. Greg hasn't been with a woman since he last saw me 6 months ago, and I can't imagine how anyone can go that long without physical contact. I've undressed him and seated him on the bed. We put the cable TV music station on, and I know I need to take it slow because he could pop in a minute. That's not what I'm after. I want him to cum at least twice. And I'm gonna try—it's kind of like a personal goal I set for myself.

11:00 p.m.: I'm in the shower now. He showered first. He is so happy and that brings me such joy—for real. Guys like Greg don't get much encouragement at being men, and to be honest, they make good little lovers because they want to please and explore and all that stuff.

11:30 p.m.: I won't let him tip the valet—I know he had to save to afford our little get together. It will probably take him another six months to be able to see me again.

11:35 p.m.: I'm in the car. Dev always worries about me on dates, even though I only see certain guys I've known for a long time. He answers on the second ring.

12:15 a.m.: Dev is in a loving mood. I love having sex with him after I see a client. It's something about giving my body back to my guy.

FRIDAY

8:00 a.m.: Dev let me sleep in. I felt him gently brush the hair from my face and kiss me softly on the cheek.

8:15 a.m.: Having coffee while Dev showers. I have one of those two-headed showers that are perfect for couples but we hardly ever shower together. I join him.

8:17 a.m.: The bastard is peeing on my leg! I try to move but now he's firing at me, so I take my shower head and blast him with cold water, and now we're just goofing around like a couple of ding-a-lings.

9:00 a.m.: I've got a bunch of emails from fans and friends wishing me good luck on my performance with a burlesque troupe tonight. I'll be working with a dozen killer-looking girls almost half my age. Dev seems real excited, and the jealousy feelings are kicking in and I hate it but I can't shake it.

9:45 a.m.: Dev is on the dance group's website. He says he's confirming the time. I'm sure he is, but I think he's checking out the hot one. I'm feeling vulnerable. He knows I'm insecure about my booty butt—I have almost a black girl booty, when all the dancers are small and tiny—and I just don't need him here right now.

12:00 p.m.: Dance rehearsal. This isn't my first time. I love the girls in the cast. They are young dancers, so fit and firm, and most have real boobies (not like mine). Dev, of course, always talks about this one girl in particular. I'm pretty sure—no, I know—that he fantasizes about her sometimes when he's having sex with me—but that's okay.

7:00 p.m.: I've showered and shaved in the guest room, because I don't want Dev looking at me naked. I've checked myself out in the mirror more in the last hour than I have in months! I guess I'm a little less secure than I thought.

9:15 p.m.: The producer says she's happy to see me and she says I look great and I'm like, "Not bad for 38!" and Dev just shakes his head. He's been saying I look great all night.

9:30 p.m.: Backstage. The girls who do have boob jobs, with all due respect, don't have the quality job I have. My boobs are famous in the XXX world. A doctor from Beverly Hills did the work and they are awesome, and they weren't cheap, either. I love showing them off to the girls—explaining how it's called a Tear Drop because the work is done above and beneath the muscle. Plus you can't see the incision.

9:45 p.m.: I'm ready to go and of course Dev is chatting with his favorite dancer. I'll admit she's hot and almost the total opposite of me. She's got long dark hair and dark brown eyes and natural boobies and she's gone to college. I'm from Minnesota who never finished high school. Plus I'm 38 years old and in my business girls are turning 18 every day. A bunch of them will be after my dollars and my fans and maybe my guy, too!

10:00 p.m.: The show starts, and I go on early for my solo number, and I rock it. Then we pull someone from the audience on stage and I get to muss him up and stuff. The show ends with this big number and of course I get a huge ovation and I just love it.

11:20 p.m.: I sign autographs and take lots of pictures and I get a lot of "You still look great," but I don't mind because I do, and "still" is not such a bad word.

1:00 a.m.: Home. I ask Dev to do me and pretend I'm the girl he likes. But Dev is no dummy—he's not biting. He says, "I just want to make love to my wife," and I say, "How about Sunset instead?" That'll do, and we have sex really aggressively and he finally rolls off and his head hits the pillow and he's out. And I'm pretty sure he was thinking about that girl the whole time.

SATURDAY

6:00 a.m.: I don't know how he does it, but Dev is up with my son and they're going to church. They go most weekends to 6:30 Mass.

6:15 a.m.: I'm in bed with my little red vibrator. I swear being alone makes me horny—maybe because I was brought up with ten brothers and sisters. I've got at least an hour and I'm lying there with my eyes shut and the ceiling fan spinning and getting myself off.

12:00 p.m.: Family day. Pizza, park, chores.

8:30 p.m.: Everyone's in bed. Dev and I are naked together but that big Sunday paper is between us—he's doing the crossword. I'm too tired to complain about the light and so I just reach over and touch his face and guess what? He takes off his reading glasses, tosses the bulky paper on the floor, turns off that lamp and cuddles with me.

The Sexy Expat Enjoying a Long-Term Marriage and a Trophy Girlfriend

29, Singapore

WEDNESDAY

6:50 a.m.: I wake up alone in a starfish pose, limbs flung toward the corners of the bed. The Husband (henceforth TH) is away on business, as he is 30 percent of the time. People assume this is hard for me, but I like my own company and the reunions are always nice. To paraphrase the writer Audrey Niffenegger, I'm glad when TH is gone, but I am always glad when he returns.

7:00 a.m.: I have a wank, barely awake and solely mechanical, no fantasy. The World Service clicks on.

7:10 a.m.: After listening to the news I make myself come again, this time thinking about Potential Trophy Girlfriend (PTG). The act is as much practical as indulgent: The extra shot of orgasm kick-starts my metabolism and I drag myself out of bed.

8:30 a.m.: I muse on PTG in the shower. "Trophy" because she is gorgeous and [cough] several [cough] years younger than me, and "potential" because neither of us wants to ask much of the other. We've had sex, but I wouldn't say we *are* having sex. Each time has been a self-contained, alcohol-driven event. She's coming over tonight to learn to bake (not a euphemism). I take the liberty of shaving my legs and putting on nice underwear.

4:50 p.m.: Hella busy afternoon at the office, punctuated by TH emailing. He's being Mr. Executive—giving speeches, going on the TV, pressing flesh—and now he's feeling small and tired and needs reassuring.

4:55 p.m.: TH is not The One, but that reassures me. Our relationship is borne of hard work rather than a thunderbolt. We have had an open relationship for six years (out of eight) and while we've always known where we'd like to be, we haven't always known if we'd get there. But for more than a year now everything has been driven by teflon-coated gears. We are communicating better than ever, we've had loads of super enjoyable group sex, and as a couple we seem to be forming something perhaps a little more substantial with another couple (PTG and Cute Boyfriend)—which is new and exciting territory.

10:10 p.m.: Baked with PTG. We accidentally-on-purpose brushed against each other, and ended up lying on the sofa together waiting for the kitchen timer to ding. And then she was gone and I was frustrated. But she went to see Cute Boyfriend—he's leaving town tomorrow so I can hardly begrudge her. Fortunately, frosting fixes most of life's ills.

10:18 p.m.: I've been thinking a lot lately of sex with PTG and Cute Boyfriend. This is a practical issue. I have slept with them both, and she has slept with TH, but we haven't had both boys naked in the same room at the same time. This is likely to happen, but I think it might freak out Cute Boyfriend. I keep meaning to sit down with him and ask what stepping-stone would make him comfortable, or where he wants to go next, but I haven't made time for that conversation yet.

THURSDAY

7:30 a.m.: Slept like I was dead—assuming that the dead have mild work-based anxiety dreams—and woke upon a World Service package about a veiled Saudi woman taking *Arab Idol* by storm. I try to put Allah out of my head as I have my morning wank. Instead I think about TH folding me in his arms and calling me a whore as he softly commands me to come.

9:15 a.m.: Beautiful statuesque Indian girl on the commuter train. She is wearing a sage green sari edged with burgundy and copper thread, and a burgundy *choli* showing a tantalizing expanse of stomach. She owns the space around her. I am captivated.

4:50 p.m.: TH emails, forlorn that he is rushing to the toilet every half hour. I ought to counter with something like "Oceans might divide us, but scatologically we are as one," (I, too, have gastro troubles), but work has pissed me off too much to want to make lame jokes.

6:00 p.m.: Thinking about sex with TH. It lurches from depressing, when we get sidelined by our jobs, to amazing when we remember that it's supposed to be fun. I often feel that our sex life lives in a box, unpacked and then swiftly repacked so we can return to asexuality. I want to receive filthy emails while I'm working, or have a hand stuffed up my top while we're alone together in a lift. But that just isn't his style.

6:05 p.m.: He also doesn't abandon himself to sex; he is always controlled and a bit distant from the process. He often counters with "They do it, too" (they don't, but it's bad form to bring up other partners, so I have to let that one go), or "It's just how I am." I'll give him that one. He always listens carefully and tries hard to respond. This is an ongoing discussion—there are times when the sex is amazing, and I remind myself that I genuinely want to be with this guy when I'm 80, sitting next to each other in bath chairs, shooting the breeze. Can't say that about anyone else I've slept with.

10:30 p.m.: PTG has just left after lesson two: chocolate fudge buttercream frosting. We have a lot of fun, sticking our faces in the bowl of melted chocolate and licking cream from each other's fingers. It's all very suggestive and very silly and then we drink beer and watch comedy and swoon over Noel Fielding in *The Mighty Boosh*. I'm not brave enough to make a move, but the excitement is fun. I feel teenaged again.

10:45 p.m.: TH and I decided to make our relationship more open after two years of failing at monogamy. The first thing we did was write a list of rules. I think there were about 12 in all, and the gist was "check first before doing anything more than kissing." My difficulty recalling them is because these days, our relationship is more organic. We needed the safety net of rules to get to a place where we naturally knew and respected each other's comfort zones.

10:49 p.m.: TH was for a long time more comfortable with me sleeping with other girls, so the first time I spent a weekend alone with Other Guy felt like a watershed moment. Other Guy is someone I met at uni and had an amazing no-strings six months of sex with. It was basically a crush that never wore off. But in the years that followed I didn't always relate to him in a way that was healthy with respect to TH. I realized I was feeling guilty about still loving him, and therefore acting furtively and defensively, so there were no parameters within which TH could feel comfortable. Since then Other Guy and I have shared a few naked weekends, which I'm very grateful for, especially because I knew he'd settle down with a proper girlfriend and she probably wouldn't be cool with him sleeping with his friends. This has since happened.

10:57 p.m.: There's sometimes sex while TH is traveling. I had the feeling that TH would be fine with the idea, so I asked, and the agreement shifted from "no sex without checking each time" to one that is more fluid: "It's fine to have sex with these people in this setting without checking first." TH sees his business trips as a chance to cut loose and pick up young ladies. I've been thrown by this when it's happened without my expecting it, but we're now at a point where I feel fine with the idea that it may or may not happen while he's away. I think the moral is that it's okay to change the status quo in small, safe increments, but if someone does something wildly unexpected, the other person is going to feel threatened and upset.

11:02 p.m.: Do we talk about sex afterward? The deal is that TH doesn't really want details, but he will get full disclosure should he ask. Most of the sex with others is in a group setting, and we tend to talk about it a lot afterward. It's a turn on. It's nice to have the connection of being in the same room having sex with other people—I can look over and know straight away that TH is happy.

FRIDAY

5:00 a.m.: Slept like a dead person until 4:00 a.m., and then slept like a wide-awake person till now. My morning wank wakes me up and warms me up, but isn't super enjoyable.

8:30 a.m.: TH arrives home while I'm in the shower. We kiss from opposite sides of the glass as if we're visiting in prison. Running late, so manage a quick chat, but am aware that I'm short changing him.

9:20 a.m.: Weird cute guy on the train. He's wearing a singlet, checkered Bermudas and leather Chucks and has shoulder-length curly hair and a goatee. Catch his eye and smile. From then on, every time I peek I catch him peeking, too.

5:40 p.m.: My work day emotions veer between frustrated, scared, angry, militant and jubilant. Decided that I will resign on Monday. The acceptance that I can walk, combined with it being Friday and TH being home has me buoyant.

9:00 p.m.: Arrive home for the grand TH reunion, and subject him to a 30-minute data dump on the work situation. Then I drag him to the bedroom for 20 minutes of fellatio and a quick shag. It feels good, necessary. TH definitely keeps me balanced. I'm feeling great.

10:00 p.m.: TH and I dance around naked to "The Prodigy" and tease each other. A sample of a new-ish drug, mephedrone, arrived in the post this week and we decide to try it out. I should point out, while I can still type, that the drug is currently legal but is unlikely to stay that way. Friends in the know describe it as somewhere between ecstasy and coke. When we were younger and living back home, we did a lot of ecstasy as it was the cheapest form of entertainment available to us, but it's been a long time.

12:20 a.m.: The mephedrone is clean. Not really like coke (affecting dopamine), more like MDMA (affecting serotonin), but milder than ecstasy. I come up gently without any big physical waves, and mostly feel floaty and chatty. TH and I talk and talk, about our life together and how our relationship has changed, our friends in London, how we relate to our families, books we've enjoyed recently, everything.

1:20 a.m.: One possibility we talk about is a permanent multiway relationship, where a third (or fourth?) party moved in with us. At this point neither of us wants that, and I suspect my life won't take that direction, but if it ever seemed viable it would certainly get plenty of consideration. This year I'd like to develop relationships with third parties that have a certain amount of emotional depth and stability, similar to that of a monogamous couple who've been dating for a short while. One poly guy I know calls this "travelling without moving," because group or secondary relationships are not necessarily heading towards the same milestones as monogamous ones, but can still develop emotionally.

2:00 a.m.: We have some floaty sex but I am starting to crash and getting ready for bed. Pop factoid: before ecstasy was made illegal, it was successfully used as a tool in some marriage guidance programs.

SATURDAY

11:20 a.m.: Ahhh, Saturday morning. No World Service, no wanking, just me and TH curled around each other.

6:30 p.m.: Post epic nap, I am heading to the mall for a massage, a bikini wax, and a haircut. Having kids is really gonna screw up my lazy weekends. I should mention that we've been trying for seven months. Initially I timed ovulation, but each month meant two weeks post-ovulation where I might've been pregnant, and getting my period felt like a loss. So we've gone back to the centuries-old method of having sex and waiting for nature to take its course. I have been *much* saner.

11:00 p.m.: Got home at ten and TH was talking to my sis on Skype. I've been missing her lovely little idiot face a lot lately. My sis knows I have an open relationship; it makes her a bit uncomfortable, but she tries hard to be accepting. I tried to come out to my mother as bi when I was about 17, and she told me that if it didn't involve her grandkids then she didn't need to know who I was sleeping with.

11:30 p.m.: My 30-year-old, hotshot executive husband just informed me that he really respects Lady Gaga as an artist, and is subjecting me to a large part of Lady Gaga's canon via YouTube. I get my revenge by making him listen to Apache Indian doing a cover of "The Israelites".

12:00 a.m.: We're talking about my birthday party. Assuming I can pull it off, I will celebrate my 30th with a private orgy. Have been to a few big, sort of commercial orgies in the past and never quite vibed with the atmosphere. Then last year I went to a private orgy and had a lovely time. So I figure I should take matters into my own hands and arrange them. We shall see if it works.

12:08 a.m.: My sex wish list: First, double penetration. This isn't a huge fantasy, but I'm certainly curious, and may get the opportunity to try it out soon. Next up is knife play. This is serious BDSM edge play. At this point Other Guy is the only person I would trust to put a blade to my skin. However, I don't think I am prepared to have the conversation where I tell TH that I want to try something hugely intimate and reasonably dangerous not with him. And finally, strap-on sex. I got one for Christmas but have yet to try it out. I have a loose agreement to try it with a girl, but every time she sees me ineptly trying to put a straw in a juice carton, she jokes that the deal is off.

12:10 a.m.: I have a pet theory that much of the way men and women relate to each other, and hence how society is structured, comes from the psychological difference between penetrating and being penetrated. So I'm very interested to see if sex feels different emotionally when I assume the role of the man.

SUNDAY

8:40 a.m.: Wake up hung over. Alcohol's aftereffects give me lots of booze-related mood swings. It was enough to make me stop drinking for a while, but drinking is a large part of my life. Work flits into my head (Sunday = practically Monday).

1:40 p.m.: Yoga, feeling much better. My dry mouth, headache, and bad mood told me to skip the class, but fortunately they were overruled by experience.

6:06 p.m.: Spend a happy afternoon at a gay pride fundraiser. Me, TH, and PTG share two bottles of champagne and get giggly and flirty, then she heads off to find Cute Boyfriend.

10:30 p.m.: I initiate sex with TH, but I'm only doing it because it's early still, and we didn't have sex yesterday. Once we get going my head catches up with my body, and both get quite carried away (fake it til you make it?). Everything started slow with the barest of butterfly touches. Appreciative noises guided onward. He ended up squeezing, pinching and pulling my nipples and clitoris—never breaking the slow pace or taking his eyes off mine. There's something about the deliberateness of that kind of intense pain that makes it incredibly hot.

11:30 p.m.: I think we both still have the remains of the mephedrone in our systems, making us more tactile and open to emotional connections. It was one of those encounters where our bodies started to flow into each other. It's definitely the most emotionally present I've been for sex since TH has returned. It was a complete communion—tuned into each other and blocking out everything else. When sex clicks for us, it really clicks.

MONDAY

7:40 a.m.: Wake, World Service, wank—you know the drill. I wank while thinking about being forced to my knees and slapped a round my face.

7:42 a.m.: I'm conscious that I haven't said much about being bisexual or masochistic. Truth is, I don't think much about these things. They are deeply and completely a part of who I am, and have been since I became sexually aware at the age of 14. I have never fought or fretted about my sexual inclinations—I just enjoy them.

7:44 a.m.: A thought on wanking in front of one's partner: I have never felt self-conscious touching myself during sex, but how I wank on my own is very different. Good old Betty Dodson's *Sex for One* helped me get past this. I mentioned to TH that a big part of my everyday life was missing, and we both agreed that we needed to masturbate more than we had been, that we were fine doing it near each other, and that it was separate from sex and we wouldn't say anything about wanting to have sex with each other. Not hiding our masturbation from each other is a good thing indeed.

7:46 a.m.: Though TH is an owl whereas I'm a lark. I get annoyed if he starts to wank just as I'm falling asleep, as the motion invariably makes me wide awake again.

7:48 a.m.: The World Service informs me that Ricky Martin is gay. This is news? Really?

9:00 p.m.: Work passes in a daze.

10:00 p.m.: TH makes sexual overtures, but I tell him I'm too tired. We remain wrapped around each other for some time.

11:15 p.m.: Snuggle up to TH and fall asleep with my head on his shoulder, holding his hand. I HATE sleeping tangled up with another person, so I think this is a sign of how much the day has thrown me off my stride.

11:20 p.m.: We've taken some massive and rewarding leaps of faith with our open relationship. My experience is that white lies or omissions can paper over the cracks for longer in a monogamous rather than a nonmonogamous relationship. Thinking about this is making me realize how completely I control my life and where it goes, and how good things are worth working hard for.

Appendix

WHAT KIND OF RELATIONSHIP IS IT?: A CHEAT SHEET

The 1500 Sex Diaries behind this book reveal that all relationships are not built equal. Each long-term couple has its own *way* of interacting, which forecasts their whole future: their sex life, friends, family, happiness, *everything*. The book refers to three relationship types: lovers, partners, and winners.

Lovers

Relationship Priorities

- Sexual exploration and fulfillment
- Intellectual or spiritual soulmate connection
- Kink or alternative lifestyle exploration
- Romance and passion
- Creative communion

These diarists prize deep emotional and intellectual honesty with their partner *right now*, and if that disappears, they often breakup. The purpose of the relationship is the connection, which they feed by interacting on many levels—emotional, spiritual, intellectual, and physical—with frequent sex.

Partners

Relationship Priorities

- Security of a life partner
- Religious partnership
- Daily companionship and hobbies
- Long-term familiarity and habit

These diarists build intimacy through shared daily activities and hobbies, and through small gestures like serving meals and greeting each other at the door. These diarists are buddies, and enjoy planning a week or month ahead, perhaps arranging next month's camping trip. Often married, these diarists frequently divorce over inattention or infidelity.

Aspirers

Relationship Priorities

- Financial security
- Professional partnership
- Lifestyle and status attainment
- Parenthood and family
- Division of labor (income, medical care, etc.)

These diarists are deep friends, bonded by shared goals that are best attained in partnership, such as growing a family, finances, or career aspirations. They are allies, in every sense of the word. These diarists think in the future, and often articulate the expectations that they want to maintain—say, "three kids, $100,000 per year, and sex twice a week." If one partner shifts goals, the relationship is threatened.

You should know that: Yes, relationships can morph from one type to another over time. And like all things in life, each type comes with great advantages and disadvantages.

The Sex Diarists

"Hands down, our sex doesn't compare with any of our past lovers. To us, that is love.*"*
35, FAULKNER COUNTY, ARKANSAS, ASPIRER

Chapter 7—Cheating: On Paper, I'm Monogamous.
In Practice...

Chapter 8—Flourishing: The More, The Merrier

Notes

Chapter 2. Soloing: I Am My Own Soul Mate
1. St. Paul: I Corinthians 7. Matthew takes a similar bent, Matthew 19:10–12.

Chapter 3. Dating: It's Simple—I Like You, You Like Me
1. Pope, Tara Parker. *For Better or For Worse: The Science of a Good Marriage,* p. 84, highlighting the research of Cindy Hazan at Cornell University.

Chapter 4. Committing: Together Forever
1. Smith, Tom W. "General Social Survey Topical Report #25: American Sexual Behavior: Trends, Socio-Demographic Differences and Risk Behaviors." University of Chicago, March 2006, p. 13. The GSS is the most accurate source of nationwide sex statistics.
2. Ibid.

Chapter 5. Recommitting: Round Two
1. Laumann, Edward. "Surveying Sex: Interview with Edward Laumann," in *Introducing the New Sexuality Studies,* edited by Steven Siedman et al., Routledge, 2010, pp. 24–25.
2. Ibid, 125.

Chapter 6. Ending: Dissonance, Breakups, Death, and Other Mishaps
1. Pope, Tara Parker. "Is It Love Or Mental Illness?" *Wall Street Journal,* February 13, 2007.

Chapter 7. Cheating: On Paper I'm Monogamous, In Practice...
1. Smith, Tom W. "General Social Survey Topical Report #25." American Sexual Behavior: Trends, Socio-Demographic Differences and Risk

Behaviors. University of Chicago, March 2006, p. 8. In 2001, *The Journal of Family Psychology* found slightly higher numbers, estimating that 20–25% of Americans will cheat during their lifetime. Unfortunately, there is little reliable data on unmarried couples.
2. Smith, Tom W., p. 21

Chapter 8. Flourishing: The More the Merrier
1. "Sex at Dawn: Why Monogamy Goes Against Our Nature," by Thomas Rogers, *Salon*, June 27, 2010.
2. Pope, Tara Parker. *For Better or For Worse*, p. 33.

Acknowledgments

Peeking into offices can be every bit as tantalizing as bedrooms, and the offices here at Sex Diaries HQ have been bustling this year, thanks to the hard work of my agent, Todd Shuster, who has believed in this project, as well as Hans Schiff and Brian Pike at CAA, and Banks Tarver at Left/Right Productions, who always knew that it belonged on the small screen. The sharp eye of my editor Tom Miller brought this volume to life, along with the support of Publisher Kitt Allan. I also thank Jorge Amaral, Laura Cusack, Richard DeLorenzo, and Matt Smollon.

The anonymous diarists, of course, deserve the bulk of the praise, for writing down their inner lives—a task in itself—and going out on a limb and *sharing* them with the world. Diarists, this is the most public thank you possible, so I thank you for sharing your lives. You are amazing people with incredible stories, and made creating this book far too much fun.

And this book would certainly not have been possible without the support of Nate Guisinger, who I am now quite certain is the best partner in the world.

Index